HEPATITIS B & C
WHAT EVERY FAMILY NEEDS TO KNOW

HEPATITIS B & C

WHAT EVERY FAMILY NEEDS TO KNOW

PAUL DESMOND

authorHOUSE®

AuthorHouse™ UK
1663 Liberty Drive
Bloomington, IN 47403 USA
www.authorhouse.co.uk
Phone: 0800.197.4150

Published by AuthorHouse 09/28/2015

ISBN: 978-1-5049-8790-5 (sc)

Print information available on the last page.

Hepatitis B & C
What Every Family Needs to Know

**A simple Risk Test & Vaccinate Manual
For Families, Occupations and GP's**

By Paul Desmond

For Dadi Janki who taught me how to -

Count honestly what I can give rather than what I can get

Have good wishes for all from a deep understanding

Care with the virtues I would want caring for myself

Contents

Abbreviations

ALT	alanine aminotransferase	a marker of liver health
BBV Nurse	Blood Borne Viral	
cHBV	chronic Hepatitis B	
FGM	female genital mutilation	
GP	general practitioner local doctor	
GUM	Genital Urinary Medicine (Clinic for sex diseases)	
HBV	Hepatitis B virus	
HCV	Hepatitis C virus	
HIV	human immuno deficiency virus	
ICU	intensive care unit	
IDU	intravenous drug user	
IVF	in vitro fertility treatment	
LFT	liver function tests	
MRSA	flesh eating superbug	
NHS	National Health Service	
NICE	National Institute of Clinical Excellence	
PEP	Post Exposure Prevention	
PHE	Public Health England	
STD/STI	sexually transmitted disease or infection	
WHO	World Health Service	

Chapter 1
Why should I get tested for Hepatitis B&C?

Just one unnoticed pin prick can transmit HBV & HCV and most of the 2 billion humans who have caught HBV & HCV did so without knowing.

It is quite fatal to imagine that a virus that infects 1 in 4 humans on Earth is for rare groups or people who do something wrong, especially when HBV is mainly silently caught by children, a billion to date and HCV is mainly silently caught by patients under anesthesia, 200 million to date.

With any virus that infects 1 in 4 humans the biggest risk is not to know how to manage it and how everyone got infected.

One hundred million of the people who have missed their HBV & HCV safety tests are expected to die of Liver Cancer or Liver Failure.

Hepatitis Screening saves lives

In the UK approximately 500,000 people with Hepatitis C, and 500,000 more with Hepatitis B are out there, 80% undiagnosed and without access to care. This equates to 1 in 65 of us in the UK living with a deadly Liver Virus, without even knowing or having a proper warning from our health service. The NHS is the only service on Earth that has not prevalenced HBV and HCV since 1995.

You may be from Africa, Asia, the Middle East or Eastern Europe and have missed your own national Hepatitis B and C test warnings by migrating here over the last 40 years like the author of this book. Or you may be an NHS patient who received organs, dialysis, surgery or a c-section in the period before hepatitis safety screening started in 1992. Or you may have travelled and received an African or Asian injection where syringe re-use is common, and millions are still infected annually. The point is, Viral Hepatitis often has no symptoms, it only has risks that need testing.

Hepatitis B & C, what every family needs to know is a book to warn the UK about Viral Hepatitis, globally approximately 200 million silent Hepatitis C infections are due to operative transfusions, inoculation and dialysis. Approximately 2,200 million people have been infected with Hepatitis B and C via contaminated blood during childhood, healthcare interventions and accidents. The point is,

Hep B or C infection is both silent and unavoidable for the vast majority of the people who get it and without a safety test it can become deadly.
The point is if more than one in 4 people on Earth have already been infected with these silent cancer causing viruses, have you been told enough about them, and more importantly about the medical, childhood, social and occupational risks that should be screened? Do you know enough about the risks of blood and forgetting to wear your plasters? Do you understand how to protect your family and yourself?

Do you have any idea how 1 in 50 Europeans got HBV or HCV infected? Do you have any idea how 1 in 60 Americans got infected? Do you know which very common infection risks you or your loved ones may have run? Do you realise that the mainly Undiagnosed Viral Hepatitis Pandemic killed one and a half million times last year, or 150 times as often as Flu? And most importantly, do you know that knowing your liver status, simply testing and adapting your diet has helped save millions of the infected from fatal consequences?

Nothing can cure a delayed safety test,

Of the army liver surgeons I've met, every single one is dealing with patients who are dying because they didn't know 21 Units of alcohol and long term hepatitis is deadly, or because they didn't know most prescriptions for pain plus hepatitis are long term deadly. Like the much missed Anita Roddick, far too many are being diagnosed needing a liver transplant they fail to receive.

Thousands have died due to simple ignorance of their infection; do not wait until symptoms that will kill you emerge to take a Hepatitis B or C test, for the at least 12 million UK citizens at high risk, it is time to test these risks and time to ensure the ones you love are also protected by Hepatitis B vaccination and by knowing their liver status.

This book lists who is recommended for Hepatitis B and C safety tests, at work, school and at home and which communities and especially children are indicated for Hepatitis B vaccination. In the UK, with up to a million already viral hepatitis infected, there are at least 10 million residents who have run NHS or Overseas Medical and Childhood Risks, risks the World Health Organisation has recommended "Safety Screening" for since 1999. Basically our unvaccinated children, workers with blood and millions arriving from Pandemic Stricken areas, our inner cities, our schools and our workplaces have simply become more infected, more undiagnosed and more infectious each year since 1995. With Hepatitis B being so infectious via blood spill also it can boom even with a cleaned up health service.

At least 600-800,000 UK residents and migrants from Pandemic areas will have livers that are long term infected and now in grave danger due to non diagnosis. The test is quick, free, painless and stops the infected accidentally destroying their livers with Common Behaviours, namely, Obesity, Alcohol, Toxic prescriptions. It is estimated up to 250,000 UK lives can be saved simply by the recommended safety screening. HBV alone has infected 60 times more people than HIV and is projected to kill 4 times the number of humans, is it sensible to not know if you have it?

This Book is configured to explain each of the main risks clearly for the millions of British citizens who have run them and now need their often life saving safety tests.

About Hepatitis B

In 2012, Public Health England Surveillance noted general patients on London wards now test 2.6% infected with Hepatitis B, while nationally patients on wards were testing at 1.6% infected with it and most worryingly our children tested 0.8% infected, a figure 35 times worse than their US counterparts!

What is Hepatitis B?

Hepatitis B is a virus that can attack the liver silently over 20-40 years, and in 10-20% of the undiagnosed cases it progresses to liver cancer or cirrhosis. Worldwide 240-350 million people have lasting Hepatitis B infection and 1,600 million have caught Hepatitis B and cleared it. In the UK 500,000 people are now lastingly infected with the virus, 80% are undiagnosed. The most common ways in which HBV is spread is via infected blood to a wound during unvaccinated childhood. One in four children in Afro Asia caught HBV before their vaccination campaigns. Further risks include unprotected sex, infected medical or street injections and many occupations that work with blood.

What happens if you got infected and are not diagnosed?

With undiagnosed HBV over 20-50 years

25% get Cirrhosis

5-10% get Liver Cancer

5-10% get Liver Failure

When diagnosed HBV

has effective medications that if necessary remove it from the blood

How is hepatitis B treated?

It is important to remember 80% of patients have a very easy to manage level of HBV virus, key to healthy life is simply to avoid toxins; especially certain long term prescriptions, alcohol and obesity. All are often harmful. The aim of therapy is to keep the Hepatitis B virus under control and to prevent any liver damage such as cirrhosis and liver cancer, excellent and effective drugs can guarantee this. In Europe, there are 1 million new infections per year due to HBV, and 14 million people long term infected with HBV. Between 24,000 and 36,000 EU deaths are attributed to HBV every year. Inexpensive Testing & Vaccination avoids these outcomes.

About Hepatitis C

In 2012, Public Health England Surveillance noted general patients on UK wards were testing 1.8% Hepatitis C infected, which again points to a boom in infection numbers due to migration and a population of 500,000 HCV infected.

What is Transfusion Hepatitis C?
Hepatitis C is a virus that can attack the liver silently over many years, and in 10-20% of the undiagnosed it progresses to liver cancer or liver failure. In 2015, there are 200 million people worldwide who are infected with this disease, 600,000 people die of HCV each year.

How Do You Become Infected?
90% of Hepatitis C was spread via health services transfusing prison blood and re using syringes, this occurred before 1992 in the West and before 2000 worldwide, thus the name Transfusion Hepatitis. 2 million UK ex patients and 10 million overseas ex patients are at risk of infection. Workers with blood, Drug injectors, maternity infections and blood spills form the rest of infections. Hepatitis C is only infectious in blood.

What happens after infection when undiagnosed?
The annual death rate is 0.3% for HCV and 0.2% for HBV after 30 years.

With undiagnosed HCV over 20-50 years results in

- 25% get Cirrhosis
- 5-10% get Liver Cancer
- 5-10% get Liver Failure

When diagnosed HCV has medications that remove it permanently

How is hepatitis C treated?
If Hepatitis C becomes long-lasting, one should discuss treatment options with their doctor. The Key to health is to avoid toxins; especially some long term prescriptions, alcohol and obesity are dangers to the HCV infected. Fortunately, the drugs are 90% effective at eradicating Hepatitis C. The aim of therapy is to eradicate the Hepatitis C virus or control the liver damage such as cirrhosis and liver cancer with lifestyle changes.

The Danger of Long Term Non Diagnosis & Delaying Testing

Would you imagine that drinking a couple of pints a day over 5 years or taking a paracetamol prescription is really odds on cirrhosis deadly?   People don't, and this is how HBV & HCV kills, it is not about drug abuse dangers; it's not even about what modern medicine may do to help.

Hepatitis is really about thousands of people who might end up down the pub with their mates, smiling like idiots, as they unwittingly destroy their livers. There is someone in every busy pub and GP Surgery in the UK doing this right now. Hepatitis is really about innocent old patients taking anti-psychotics with their frail long term silently hepatitis infected livers and dying.

- **For the initial 10-20 years hepatitis is dormant and very little liver damage (high alts) occurs in the majority of patients**

- **During the next 10 years a gradual damage is seen with fibrosis (permanent liver scarring) beginning in 40% of patients**

- **However at 20-30 years toxins, such as alcohol and paracetamal silently speed liver destruction many times over until fatalities occur**

After about 30 years, especially if you are using common prescriptions (page 124), the liver will fully scar and start to fail, leading to de-compensation of the liver or liver cancer. Basically, it is expected 10%-15% of the undiagnosed infected will die. Large portions of the newly diagnosed in the UK are at the cirrhosis and three hundred times the cancer risk stage and had no idea they were ill. Our big problem is when hundreds of thousands of people are long term unknowingly infected, and our culture is unwarned or tested and cheap alcohol flooded, ever more obese and "binge" medicating.

The most dangerous thing about these viruses is their ability to infect silently and slowly over decades, just as silently send your health into a fatal spin while you still feel well.

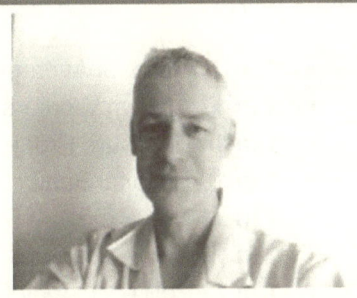

Is your job killing you?

Every year thousands of people, including the retired from the professions below, make a simple mistake; they take medicines or socially drink with their undiagnosed Viral Hepatitis B & C, many liver damage and die as a result.

Viral Hepatitis is a unique Pandemic, very often intelligent Doctors and Nurses are on the helpline finding they themselves are ill or dying due to poor screening and being ignorant of their liver status. All these roles below are recommended for vaccination and safety testing.

Nurses	Carers	First Aiders
Morticians	Tattooists	Soldiers
Sports people	Cleaners	Police & Security
Hairdressers	Sanitation	Dental Assistants
Beautician/Botox/Wax	Custodial Staff	Lab Technicians
Emergency Workers	Sex Workers	Porters
Caretakers	Special Needs	Prosthetics
Overseas Workers	Fosterers	Funeral Staff
Chefs, Builders, Mechanics,	& Glaziers (wounds)	Doctors

"All employees have a right to wait until full HBV vaccination is completed and proof of immunisation for hepatitis b is provided before starting works that are a risk of infection." Green Book on Immunisation, Department of Health 2015.

Both HBV and HCV have excellent treatments. We are in an era where it is much better to know about an infection. The concern is the bulk of staff who work with blood and are still unvaccinated for HBV and never tested for Hepatitis B & C throughout their careers, this is all too true of teacher, carer, cleaner, security and beautician staffs"

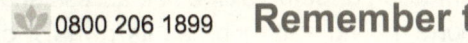 0800 206 1899   **Remember to ask your doctor**

The Extent and Reality of Occupational HBV Infections

Below Medical Studies show how often different Public Occupations caught HBV before HBV vaccination became mandatory in the 1990's.

- **1 in 38** National Average   Tedder et al 1989.
- **1 in 17** Asylum Workers   Holt et al 1985.
- **1 in 14** Exposure Prone Health Workers Fagan et al 1987.
- **1 in 19** Hospital Staff   Vandervelde et al 1985.
- **1 in 31** Non Exposure Prone Health   Smith at al 1987.
- **1 in 10** Crime Scene Officers   Morgan-Capner et al 1988.
- **1 in 22** Police Custody Officers   Morgan-Capner et al 1988.

What is immediately clear to the reader is just how much these employees caught HBV! With HBV tripling in prevalence in many workplaces since 1990 most workers with blood in the private sector and even public employees are still wholly unvaccinated or partially vaccinated for HBV.

Unfortunately low pay and zero hours staff, especially carers, cleaners, health and teaching assistants, security guards, nominated first aiders, child contact sports, beauticians, nursery and foster staff and trainees all seem to be far less vaccinated than is required. Many employers have no idea of the risk and many have been very misled by NHS information as it stands online. Few health and safety departments understand HBV and HCV infections are from blood spill and have happened 2000 million times already, many still think sex and drugs are the common transmission routes.

Running the National Hepatitis B Helpline over 6 years we have dealt with thousands of staff at risk, most of who have really struggled to get good advice or even a vaccine they can afford. There have also been hundreds of infections among all of the Industries, with sadly many deaths to report. New groups noted reporting infections are chefs, climbers, glaziers, hajis, FGM girls, insulin families, amateur boxers and rugby players, builders, eczema and cutical cut patients, the army who visit prisons, hospitals, counselors from lawyers to priests, specialists in wheel chairs, replacement hips, surgical gowns and most worryingly schools..

Having advised on 300,000 plus occupational HBV vaccinations, certain key issues need raising. With each infection or outbreak we risk access and cross reference all other Industry reports, noting each job has its own list of risks and transmission routes and how Companies, Schools and many GP's are giving completely different and often quite incorrect guidance.

Hepatitis B & C Occupational Disease Facts

- HBV infects 1.6% and HCV 1.8% of patients on UK wards
- HBV is so infectious, 3 pricks stained with hbv blood means infection
- HBV & HCV infections 95% happen silently.
- HBV infects 350 million incurably and 2 billion passingly
- HBV & HCV silently over 50 years kill 15% of the infected
- HBV is expected to kill 90 million people
- HBV Vaccine has been used safely on 2 billion newborns and staff

All Workers with blood need vaccinations and safety testing

Any job role that involves contact with blood is a real risk. Many, many retail staff from beauticians to cleaners, from barbers to dental assistants, from store security to store first aid person, from funeral parlours to massage parlours, Most are not taught enough about blood hygiene and the risks from viral hepatitis clearly, many have no idea of their risk at all.

Even many general public jobs asylum carers and teachers may be regularly dealing with blood or at risk of assault, without the correct information regarding blood hygiene and HBV vaccination. Very few such workers realise blood is infectious in one in sixty five UK citizens, very few realise blood to wound is a hundred times more potentially infectious than a one night stand with someone HBV positive and finally even fewer have been made aware undiagnosed viral hepatitis is a decimating silent carcinogen. It's time we all understood Viral Hepatitis infected blood is infectious to open wounds and 1 in 12 human beings bleed such blood. We need to get the hang of our premiership blood hygiene as well as our condoms, quick.

Systems are broken, in all our Supermarkets a £1000 is often spent privately HBV vaccinating the 3 Chemists, yet the same money could have protected the 20 first aiders, security guards and cleaners at far greater risk of violence and accident if spent in house on vaccinating all at risk. Councils, Prisons and many major employers waste millions on expensive private vaccinations they could do themselves at 10% of the cost. Far too few staff who deal with blood have read their right below before commencing work

"All employees have a right to wait until full HBV vaccination is completed and proof of immunisation for Hepatitis B is provided before starting works that are a risk of infection." Green Book on Immunisation, Department of Health 2015.

NHS Doctors and Specialist Calls to the Helpline

Liver Specialist Zambian
Called as his two old medical college surgeons had recently died from HBV liver cancers and he had no idea of his vaccination status, just 44.

Doctor
Tested positive overseas has never notified the NHS, stressed does no exposure prone work, called due to advancing liver disease.

Dentist
His Practice has overlooked Hepatitis B Vaccination boosters and immunity testing for decades, common problem, sent Vaccination Pack.

Dentist tested HBV positive
Did not know treatment could save his career Dental Council have no retrench plan for infections, contacted Dental Council.

NHS Radiographer tested HBV positive
Caught HBV in childhood thought went away, now refused as a radiographer tests indicated she's chronic and infectious, arranged referral.

Audiologist tested HBV positive years after vaccination
Was quitting career talked her round. Poor woman was told to see GP about her results and ended up stalking liver doctors at a hospital.

Midwife
Undetectable on Entacavir needs an NHS post diagnosed by new post Just great to have a simple care path for him Makes we think of all the staff who have been diagnosed after starting work and marched off by security.

Psychiatrist/Therapist
Needed guidance on working with asylums and prisons, mailed custodial pack. Sent olive book and Royal College of Nursing have stuff too. Said her right to work there is fine but the prejudice has often been seen it's like literally some prisons and asylums are all vaccinated and some are hardly at all. I'm still hearing about gloves and Post Exposure Prevention is the rules like its good from units.

NHS Doctors and Specialists

Prevalence. HBV infects 1.6% and HCV 1.8% of patients on UK wards

Transmission Routes
With half the health service now from nations where at least half the people catch HBV, doctor infections seem confined to childhood, training and failing immunity risks.

Risk Assessment
In 2001 a study of 10,000 UK NHS staff showed 1.4% of surgeons and 1% of physicians had HCV and huge numbers are untested for HBV.

Deaths
The youngest report was 43 which is far too young for a doctor. The eldest was 90 and it seems a generation of elders is missing testing on retirement.

Fallacies. Poor HBV / HCV testing of doctors is not fatally dangerous for them

UK Hospital Consultants, Surgeons and General Practitioners are given very patchy and often outdated information about Hepatitis B and C in general. In training sessions 40% are unaware of their HBV Vaccination Immunity levels. With Hepatitis C all staff accessed testing in 2000 and the 1% infected were cared for, however with the far more common and infectious hepatitis b no testing has been done in many cases. We get numerous calls from staff diagnosed when changing Trusts, we get calls from staff infected as immunity wears off, calls from staff that never attained immunity and calls from staff that had HBV in the first place but were vaccinated without testing.

There is a huge variable between Trusts at reading HBV results, we had a Surgeon mentioning the worst month of his life as his core anti body was investigated and security removed him from the hospital "like he had Ebola". There is also a variable on the treatment of the newly diagnosed staff and little guidance on making the HBV or HCV rapidly undetectable. Calls relating to leaving the profession or avoiding testing are testament to that.

Junior Doctors are often shattered by a HBV or HCV diagnosis, it seems better to test and vaccinate at the outset, senior doctors often have failed immunity scores and retired doctors are often denied boosters. With doctors an atmosphere of fear is created every time a doctor is marched off the premises for having HBV or HCV and safety testing is simply avoided.

NHS Nurse Calls to the Helpline

Ghanaian Nurse
Diagnosed November has appointment to see a specialist in July. Poor woman has suffered terribly from NHS choices. Explained what an inactive low risk infection is and also how she will manage, awaiting her bloods, it is just awful people are left with "100 times more infectious than HIV" and "often creates liver cancer" and no job or pay for 9 months.

Ex Nurse
Ill tired and needs help very poor understanding of her HBV everything has kind of convinced her career and life is over. Wept when she understood the meds and vaccine Nurses can fall out of care way too quickly.

Nigerian Nurse
Tested positive on changing hospitals this is getting such a common call Cruel HR marched her out of the building and new job on hold GP doubled agony by refusing Tenofovir Sent to Graham foster and career back on track. As the nurse noted how many just give up? Well we have heard from a few.

Remploy African nurse wants to do care but is HBV+ Explained meds and non infectious Good to see his career can continue many give up

Nigerian nurse
Low load had kids and husband no onward infections just diagnosed at work had been working for years after 3 shots and no titer

Pilipino Nurse
Can he declare his status and get a job in UK. Explained yes and found out he is a nurse here already, explained with meds he can practice, astonishment tears every Chinese/ Pilipino is like this. Hundreds of HBV nurses have downloaded our work for the NHS page, yet none have been noted arriving!

Nurse Cut foot in Majorca on romantic break and mentioned her HBV in casualty boyfriend got first plan home. Emerges she has been told at work low to undetectable risk so carry on. Several months down the line the man and his lovely nurse are married and boy

Nurse called she goes to Malaysia for HBV meds, I said get them here free and put undetectable on your NHS file save £8000 per year she said no.

NHS Nurses Issues

Risk Assessment
In 2001 a study of more than 10,000 NHS staff showed 1% of Nurses positive for HCV, however there has never been a comprehensive screening for HBV and huge numbers are still untested for HBV

2015 Prevalence HBV infects 1.6% and HCV 1.8% of patients on UK wards

Access. Many Nurses are insufficiently HBV vaccinated & HBV titre tested

Transmission Nurses report poor needle stick and post exposure care. We have had so many calls related to these, we have developed a role play training we want in the Nurse Curricula. Nurses have a right to know their wards are 7 times more infected with HBV and HCV than the PHE guesstimate, we are 3.5% infected rather than 0.5% and 1 in 29 is a lot more than 1 in 200.

Deaths In the US it is known a Nurse dies daily from HBV here it is not. Again this needs to be in the Nurse Curricula.

Fallacies Nurses are safe without rigorous HBV/HCV testing and titre testing

Nurse
Returned after career break without a booster and caught acute HBV. She is in King's ICU. Her partner is in bits, transfusion even survival is the situation.

Nurse retired
HCV infected Charing Cross 1980 no referral or compo since. GP binge and parked medicating without liver insight. Nitro spray, monsorib, adizem, ramipril, asprin, bandroflumethizide, ventolin, rusanastaline, omprazole.

Nurse retired
HBV for 35 years and now liver cancer, this Nurse from Harrow was just so serene. Their selflessness earns better care than this one just had, never had a soul to talk to, got her referred and made her understand the can't cope, exhaustion, confusion is coming from her awful liver scores"

Every Nurse should know about HBV and the value of diagnosis and immunity testing. Two of the Nurses above died while we compiled this book.

Carer, First Aid, Porter, Health & Dental Assistant Helpline Calls

St John HBV Infected 1992 flatlined during liver cancer surgery 2014.

St John HBV positive Another volunteer unable to get a jab caught HBV and infected partner, in dialogue with St John

First aid instructor and policewoman had never heard of some HBV risks or its prevalence, explained blood hygiene and how in 1990 1 in 17 crime scene officers had acute HBV signs sent Info and want to liaise

Carer HBV positive
Great Ormond Street Nursery Carer infected after 18 months via cutical cuts

Carer HBV positive
Nigerian dementia terminal carer for years, not even trained right in gloves and scrubs, been alone since diagnosis 08 only referred recently due to healthy results this poor man basically thought he had HIV not HBV, common.

Porter HBV Positive
Worked unvaccinated on surgery wards with severe hand eczema

Care home worker worked with HBV positive patient shaving changing wounds etc unvaccinated for 14 months employers thought vaccination unnecessary asked employee to pay if he is worried, common.

Care home Worker laid off for not cleaning HBV wounds unvaccinated!

Care home 5000 poorly and unvaccinated staff in care homes, 60% African staff all untested. Arranged quote feel cost will delay forever again.

Care home unvaccinated staff doing exposure prone, again management resistance GP has already said unnecessary

Care home another company talking about HBV like its vaccine has just been discovered

Carer Needle stick
Care home unvaccinated and exposure prone work! Got vaccinated developed Carer Vaccination Pack

Carers, First Aiders, Porter, Health & Dental Assistants

2015 Prevalence HBV infects 1.6% and HCV 1.8% of patients on UK wards

Costs
Act as a tremendous break on HBV vaccinations at £300. It is a month's rent for these staff, then again companies with 50 staff face £15,000 costs and often pre and post test counseling needs. Things are further complicated by Consent Forms and their usage and by huge GP and Chemist variables of advice, care and cost. We as a nation send millions of these jabs as Aid at £5 a course overseas and yet millions are charged a prohibitive £300 plus here.

Access To care is massively affected by some GPs saying needed and some not needed, some saying free and some charging £300. So many Care Homes we have to explain, "No it is not from heroin and for addicts it is from blood and for you!" Quite simply millions are getting partial or zero warnings or pitiful access to information.

Risk Assessment
Far too many staff are simply read NHS information that says 1 in a 1000 and exposure prone only. The least paid, the least educated about the risks tend to face them the most, many risks are ignored and influenced by cost, many staff are never tested or vaccinated, most managers receive mixed advice. We have had 8 confirmed reports of child first aiders catching HBV, in particular endemic community children are doing first aid without HBV vaccinations and therefore getting infected.

Transmission Routes Staff with cutical, eczema and work cuts catch HBV rapidly. Sharps injuries, assaults, spills must be presented as unavoidable. Nominated First Aiders are often 5 years away from training when called to act; few have access to gloves and scrubs or viralcides.

Deaths
      Carer End stage HBV, worked with blood for years in Home caught HBV in 1978. With ascite's draining and blood everywhere, a nightmare way to die, Sent info and lots good wishes, died.

Falsehoods Many employers assume infections never happen or can be helped by post exposure activities, a fatal approach to a silent infector and killer.

Tattooist, Piercer, Hairdresser, Beauticians Helpline Calls

MP Stephen Pound Infected with HBV at a high street tattooist, cleared

Tattoo infection Teenager had tattoo 8 weeks before, I visited the parlour, inspected chronic filth. Explained **cross contamination** events I had seen, blood on till, blood on her face, blood on clothes and she rubbed the client's blood on her eyebrow stud, she said "She doesn't believe in vaccinations." Or seemingly any sort of client safety, called Police and Council, zero reactions.

Piercing Infection 3 and 6 month babies chronically infected with HBV, the HBV was still on piercing gun when symptoms emerged 3 weeks later.

Bridal Asian Woman Had beauty prep for wedding in India Botox parties, lipo, tattoos or piercings, all possible risks, HBV infection, wedding was off.
Acute Tattoo infection Man had two tattoos about 8 weeks ago, unable to trace parlour, we need desperately to create national response path

Tattoo infection Lady had eye brow colored in 2002 in room in Rumania, went through our HBV mom training and now wants to help other moms. Has actually cleared hbv naturally She asked if eye brow threading was safe. I've watched the girls tongue abrading and rubbing away and yes, unsafe.

Scratcher Tattooist Started in prison with a needle, bought tattoo and piercing equipment later, opened a shop, barely realized one patient can infect another! He is good at sounding hygienic without 95% of the medical facts.

Northern Beauty College Beautician Her college trainer had found it impossible to arrange or advise on HBV vaccination in Yorkshire, her College has run for years without good information or a vaccine capability. Sent Pack
London College and Surburban College Beauty tech and no vaccinations, hundreds left to try to understand how and if a vaccination is necessary, will try to visit to educate and vaccinate them all

Excellent Piercing Hygienist Poz Piercer Body Mod Artist, developed dental clean safety for clients at his Scarz & Barz Studio at 01473 255 857 and can be called for advice pre piercing. Guides our ban the Piercing Gun Campaign

Excellent Tattoo Hygienist Rick Stevens President of the Tattoo and Piercing Union helped develop the Tattoo & Piercing UK Safety Toolkit. Hygiene advice, Rick himself and Toolkits are at http://www.tpiu.org.uk

Tattooist, Piercer, Hairdresser and Beautician Issues

Prevalence HBV infects 1.6% of patients and HCV 1.8% on NHS wards

Risk Assessment The Blood Bank does not accept clients for a year after a piercing or tattoo as HBV and HCV infections from the tattoos and piercings can take many months to show up. So in 2015 the only organisation that tests clients for HBV and HCV after their procedures is telling us they regard the tattooed or pierced in the UK as infectious as those having unprotected sex. Sadly the Industry does have excellent dental clean parlours and the correct training in the Tattoo and Piercing Tool Kit, but there is no enforced training of it or mandatory HBV vaccination of the staff in this highest risk profession. In the wrong hands Tattoo & Piercing Guns are very deadly weapons. If you have ever done anything outside a dental level of hygiene, especially in an unlicensed parlour or at a home, even if you feel well, get HBV and HCV Tested now. A bad tattooist will say clean needle and inks with a flourish, a good one can explain how everything you can see is sterile, and how it stays that way, including most importantly himself. He will be a HBV vaccinated cross contamination expert. He will know every place his gloves touch.

Costs The £150-300 HBV vaccination cost acts as a tremendous break on HBV vaccinations. This disaster is worsened by GP and Chemist variables.

Needs - Think before you Ink!
Excellent Tattooist and Piercer Hygiene Champions need enshrining
Poz Piercer and the Tattoo Union Rick Stevens can be contacted first
Least cost vaccinations and tests for clients and Artists
Real risk data for clients and Artists from blood bank
Free meds and career guarantee for infected tattooists and staff
HBV Vaccination enabled parlours
Outbreak Control national hotline with action team
Moving from a British Standard to a Corgi Type System
A Premiership Blood Hygiene module in Schools
Banning unlicensed gun sales and practitioners and piercing guns
Awareness Days revealed huge numbers of graduates in a booming array of beauty courses were unvaccinated for HBV as they begin work. They are quite untrained in dental levels of blood and cross contamination hygiene.

Transmission Routes cross contamination hygiene is behind most infections. **Fallacies**. Imagining a new needle is safety, when there are 50 more precautions. Imagining the Industry is safe without rigid training and inspecting

Plumber, Caretaker & Cleaner Helpline Calls

Plumber Male
Really ill caretaker, wife convinced he has cheated, spoke to wife lots blood spill at school only he cleans it good understanding now, subsequently died.

Cleaner
Picked up HBV from his work constant hand cuts and cleaning blood GP decided his gay partner the cause so they split up but partner had cleared HBV 4 years earlier. Sad misunderstanding but talked it through he rang ex and apologized, sad people and often clinicians jump to these conclusions

Cleaner Bar Maid
Asked clear up broken bloody glass, cut caused HBV.

Cleaner Surrey Council
2 week delay in PEP boss sent to chemist instead of having plan for A & E. Common, advised test and sent blood hygiene info and green olive books must add both to website front page added Cleaners Pack

Plumbing Waste Sewage Company Audit
Across the company seems that hundreds are unvaccinated and many have poor English. There is not an understanding of plasters and it seems gloves and even boots in sewers leak. Road sweepers may miss gloves or masks with dust pan and brush sweeping up pan spit. Concerningly, many workers did not know wounds hoover up HBV in sewers.

African Is contract cleaner and doorman no vacs or risk from GP? The GPs who don't vaccinate private employees seem to advise poorly on HBV risk

Worker Cleans operating theatres and is unvaccinated for years arranged Employer very keen to learn vaccinated 50 staff

Nurse How do you clean with blood? Not sure which cleaning fluids to use and just how important are gloves with wounds. One of my first calls in 2010.

Albanian Cleaner on my doorstep with flight luggage said he read the website and God said we can save him and had flown in. Arranged the long range get a London Bridge Specialist and do treatment anywhere in EU with annual checks. He is doing fine and visits every year!

26

Plumbers, Caretakers & Cleaners

Prevalence HBV infects 0.8% and HCV 0.9% of the general public

Costs

There are again ridiculous levels of variation in price, the zero hours staff run the greatest risks and get the worst advice. At £300 the vaccine is almost unused, even marigold gloves that hole in minutes are costed 3 pairs a week. Cleaning companies are not good at the £15,000 sudden outlay for 50 staff; incidents of very poor third party advice from consultants in the vaccine business are common.

Access

In many smaller companies very few cleaners are able to access any kind of risk information about blood at all, when we remember HBV has infected 1 in 4 humans already and they were not cleaning blood, this ignorance can be seen as fatal. This is worsened by the language and cost barriers.

The latest fads in larger companies include recommending a vaccine shot after exposure when it is useless by hospitals and schools, to offering the option of vaccination with a list of reasons why it is unnecessary by an Autistic School in an endemic community.

Risk Assessment & Transmission Routes

With cleaning we have found the infected cleaners and plumbers teach us a lot about transmission as we go along. Bloody glass is "sharps" dangerous and we get enough calls from the infected that clean it, right down to Bradford Glaziers being more infected than most.

Hand wounds during cleaning just occur, bleach cracks, eczema, cutical cuts, all are rarely monitored and controlled infection gateways. The equipment is often wrong, latex gloves and rationed marigolds are zero protection for a cleaner! Clip action draw string tampon bins need gloves also. The knowledge that Pooh and sewage can be highly HBV and HCV infectious is needed. Underground workers need plasters and viralcides on them.

Deaths As a cirrhotic plumber put it "If blood is the new asbestos people who work with it should know."

Fallacies. Many employers assume these silent infections never happen

Police, Security Helpline Calls

Detective Constable retired, caught HBV on the job has had a transplant requests safety tests for all retiring officers

Detective Constable Keith Mole
Keith was stabbed as an officer in 1980. His life saving transfusion gave him HBV as was very common back then. After his infection until retiring Keith was NOT referred to an expert doctor by his GP so he developed liver cancer. He has now had half his liver removed and is concerned hundreds of thousands of security staffs are at risk of this cancer causing virus many retired staff also, all are unaware and untested for HBV & HCV.

Seven Community Support policeman out of eight not vaccinated
Complex procedures at GP many told no risk arranged Police Pack and Metropolitan Intranet Payment method

Policeman HBV Infected covered in blood from drug addict and no HBV vaccination, his immuno compromised panicking partner needs accelerated course and condoms for 8 weeks calmed

Police Wife Partner just diagnosed acute, ex police now security guard, missed his vacc somehow. She's in tears waiting her results, why does nobody give these people info (printed)

Security Guard Sent stabbed guard for test for his HBV risk, then refused a HBV vaccination as he is not deemed at risk, this is "normal" in Supermarkets.

Security Guard Big drop in virus co incides with a liver friendly lifestyle

Security Guard Recent infection not trained in blood hygiene thought had HIV Sent referral letter explained could clear did not know this

Doorman Positive Seems like no job mentions the risk of blood at the get go

Doorman Diagnosed and told no babies why do GP's say this? Just amazed at these reports being common feel what is said is big danger for baby and then no babies is "heard"

Homeless charity 5000 staff unvaccinated for 20 years advised tracking

Police & Security Staff Issues

Prevalence
HBV infects 1.6% of patients and HCV 1.8%, however from the extremely localized support police and security standpoint the key is the level of infection in the community they serve. 10% is Africa and Far East. Eastern EU, the Middle East and Asia are 3%. This is where many officers work.

Costs
Another case of the closer to the criminal or community or blood risk the less the awareness and budget for HBV vaccination or HBV and HCV testing. The majority of door securities are still unvaccinated and cost is a major culprit.

Access
To care is also frustrated by a complete lack of awareness of risk. Many security staff has a Gym background wherein ignorance of blood hygiene and usage of steroids is common. Immigration, Court Services and detention officers are also victims of very varied regional practice.

Risk Infection Assessments
It is noted that with HBV, HCV and HIV, the infected prisoners often know exactly how to infect enemies with their viruses in fights instantly.
Infected Officer, 3 pricks from bloody sharp,
Infected Officer, blood transfused with a single bite,
Infected Warder, blood spat in the eye.

With 26,000 incidents of aggression noted on Mental Health wards alone the scale of violence faced by staff becomes clear also.
10 rounds and the International Boxing Federation notes HBV will transmit to an opponent. David Haye refused 20 million to fight a HBV positive Russian. This would be a statistically normal risk for a London Doorman's Career.

Transmission Routes
Arrest   Decent gloves could prevent many infections.
Crime Scene   Blood to rubber glove, glove to radio, radio to shaving cut.
Custody   Which handcuff is yours officer?

Deaths Unless tested for HBV and HCV officers will continue to die

Fallacies. Many employers simply assume the infections never happen

Teacher, Special Needs, Nursery, Fosterer & Custodial Calls

Mum
Son bitten in urban special need school, GP denied HBV vaccination and risk, common problem, only the UK denies these kids. Mum vaccinated in Poland.

Birmingham Secondary Principal advised that she may have 6 (high viral load) children at school, admitted she had already caught HBV from a pupil.

Nursery Worker Caught HBV from doing the first aid or a teething toddler bite

Prison officer Went to 12 GPs and Chemists, no HBV vaccination, there is no networking, the prison not allowed to use prisoners vaccines in own fridge.

Bradford School 80% Migrant children special needs staff all unvaccinated

Council Lost entire HBV vaccination record for borough and need to revaccinate from start several thousand staff unbelievable, they chose a £400 por Vaccination Company naturally. They could have managed to vaccinate every child in Hackney as well for the money

Autism Worker Recommended the post accident option? Not told that HBV is 10 times more common in their communities than it was. Not told that 3 bites or scratches and infections are probable and definitely not told that vaccination is the EU mandatory norm in their profession. 3,000 staff.

Language school Has placed thousands of Chinese who come to learn English with families who have kids all untested and unvaccinated. Did not feel things would change

Afghani Boy Although told HBV is a sex disease he never understood it is a blood virus has been fostered with some 50 people over 10 years he also played pokey with a compass at school for two terms key worker and boy horrified and facebooked all contacts with test advice The whole fostering industry is just off the planet

Teacher read a HBV infected toddler teething bite is a 3 to 1 risk of infection for HBV, while sex with a HIV positive adult is a 800 to 1 risk of HIV.

Explained it is very true, not a typo.

Teachers, Special Needs, Custodial Fosterers, Nursery Issues

Prevalence
HBV infects 0.8% of child patients and HCV 0.4%, however from the extremely localized teacher childcare standpoint the key is the level of infection in the community they serve. Africa and Far East are 10%, Eastern EU, the Middle East and Asia are 3%. This is where many teachers work.

Costs
Another case of the closer to the community or blood risk the less the awareness and budget for HBV vaccination or HBV and HCV testing. The majority of nominated first aiders, special needs staff are still unvaccinated and cost is the major culprit.

Access
To care is also frustrated by a complete lack of awareness of risk. Many teaching staff has local education authority guidance for little or zero plasters and no background wherein blood hygiene is common. We find HBV positive orphans need low risk info on file and our HBV mom pack to offer prospective parents to increase adoption rates. Not a single teacher in the UK seems aware a billion children have had HBV already!

Risk Assessment
Children present with serious risks until 11 and get infected the most during those years. Teething, Scratching, Biting, Falling over, Poking and even help Poohing are all normal behaviours and therefore garanteed risks here. The calls below regarding HBV infections especially are constant on the helpline
- School first aider infected by a pupil bleed onto her scratch
- Nursery carer at Great Ormond carer infected via cutical cuts
- Nursery carer caught HBV from a toddler blood spill
- School care taker caught HBV from the blood spills
- 18, did St John first aid no vaccination her and partner HBV infected
- Teaching Assistant reported sharp milk teeth as a transmission route
- 16, asked to clean up blood, caught cHBV, is a qualified doctor now.
- 17, asked to porter with hand eczema touched blood now acute HBV
- A Principal advised of 6 carriers already had caught HBV from a pupil

Deaths Are 10 to 30% of the undiagnosed **Fallacies** Many perhaps most simply assume Schools and Special School HBV outbreaks are not common.

31

Trainees, Overseas Workers, Sex Workers Calls

Trainee Manager Dentistry
Head of infection control has sent out trainees all unvaccinated and seldom titer tested. Imagine if bike riders took 9 months to get untested helmets on.

Trainee Nurse HBV positive referred to occupational health

Trainee 16 year old girl cleaning toilets got HBV infected and admitted acute

Chef Greece just diagnosed panic never heard of HBV got his mum to ring had child vacs from 95 that failed now. Why do we export unvaccinated chefs to endemic areas? Sent acute info reassured.

Chef Thailand Regular cuts zero hygiene in busy kitchen a real like manic Ramsey Manager Seriously ill with no help over there mum sending money to get him home Why do we send so many unvaccinated to these places?

Chef's wife Infected chef hubby working with all African eastern EU kitchen and constant wounds unplastered found others in kitchen with HBV after restaurant did screening and vacs am convinced we have another transmission route

Porter 17 year old Acute infection after 3 months working in a hospital no other risk, poor info from GP, explained recovery plan for acute patients.

Dozens of Nurse Trainees Working one month no vaccination boss not paying GP offered 6 month course Tired of this asked to work before immune common create flyer of green book rules needed

Sex Worker Vietnamese boy of 15, trafficked and infected.

Gay Rent Boy Checking his vaccination is sufficient protection for cum in the eye and vigorous anal sex, said yes and gave up on sandwiches.

Prostitutes Union Rumanian girl HBV undetectable on meds and yes safe for all services!

Prostitutes Union Still girls working unvaccinated and still no sign of blow job transmission

Trainees, Overseas Workers, Sex Workers

Prevalence
Huge numbers travel to work overseas with no idea they are onward to a nation where 95% of people get HBV or the transmission routes. Many also do not know the UK general public levels of HBV and HCV are booming.

Costs
As so many trainees are at the outset of their careers they are at their poorest, this often delays or forgets the issue. Overseas workers are often advised wrongly to not be vaccinated even when onward to Afro Asia!

Access
Ignorance of risk and prevalence causes a large number of staff to miss their protections. Many advisors, GP's, Travel Agents, and Employers forget to vaccinate. Many are told they are not planning sex or drugs so they do not need vaccination, even health tourists and children are denied!

Risk Assessment
Trainees by their nature are least skilled and most accident prone in their first 6 months and this is often when vaccinations are missed. This is very emotive for medical, aviation many careers, between 16 and 19 we get many calls regarding infections at work. Large numbers of sex workers are from endemic regions and many have no GP's, trafficked sex workers, especially boys are often very infected.

Transmission Routes
Overseas workers catch HBV from healthcare often, no overseas doctor consulted imagined they would be unvaccinated. Chinese martial artist travelers, Gap Year Students, English Teachers, even Aid workers forget. Sexually speaking after years of callers and prostitute feedback there is no report of oral sex infecting anyone. Massage parlours and a whole range of touch therapies also have no training in blood hygiene or HBV vaccination.

Deaths
Overseas often the easiest place to get HBV is the hardest place to get help for it.

Fallacies. Many employers simply assume the infections never happen

Lab Staff, Prosthetics, Morticians, Soldiers & Emergency Calls

Company manufacture hip replacements Two infections and decided to vaccinate everyone Taught vaccination to them arranged least cost supply

Employer Has many staff fitting prosthetic limbs forgot boosters, got too nervous to stay on line, when realised staff were at poss risk Very coy poor understanding would not give email Doubt she knows enough to protect her staff is busy protecting her liabilities

Blaser Mills Unvaccinated lawyers in prisons often have never heard of hepatitis Sent custodial carer pack

Working couple Washes surgical gowns unvaccinated for years did not understand an open wound could infect him Arranged privately as company not interested

Hospital Worker Has HBV and Noted anti HDV on his London hospital report went into panic unable to get through to secretary and he works at the hospital Explained HDV is common extra infection along with HBV. Explained it responds well to treatment and he will be fine know hospital well and arranged help group meeting.

Biochemist Did test but took GP 7 months to tell him HBV positive with terrible information. Made him patients advocate hopefully for NICE.

Ambulance Para Medics & Fireman We take numerous calls from private company staff who are unvaccinated and even have had GP's state no risk.

Ex SAS
Cleared HBV infection in army US troops gob smacked he was not vaccinated. Pitiful GP info mentioned HBV carrier to his insurance co when he is HBV immune, explained he is not infected or permanently damaged, GP told him HBV can come back later in life. Amazing, healthiest caller ever and he was refused life insurance due to GP saying a cleared infection is a active one.

Lab Staff, Prosthetics, Morticians, Soldiers & Emergency Issues

Prevalence

HBV infects 1.6% of patients and HCV 1.8%

Costs Again complete profit madness sees private companies charging up to £400 a vaccination. Many prosthetics and funerary staff are still unvaccinated and cost is a major culprit.

Access

Ignorance of risk and prevalence causes a large number of staff to miss their protections. Many advisors, GP's, Employers forget to vaccinate. Numerous troops needed US vaccinations in Gulf War One, since then almost none of the veterans have been properly tested. Private ambulance companies often have unvaccinated and unwarned staff.

Risk Assessment

Had a mortician with a sissor stick from a HBV source. It chronically infected him with HBV. That is the point with all this, just 3 pricks and you are infected.

Transmission Routes

We have noted HBV infections as commonly from routes where there is no pain eg the blood sample is handled often, handling slides, cabinets, equipment in labs with old cuts or conditions eczema etc as from with impact sharps from a surgical tray.

Deaths

Staffs call at about 50 diagnosed with cirrhosis quite often, as with many poorly vaccinated professions the HBV and HCV safety testing is usually atrocious too.

Fallacies.

Many employers simply assume the infections never happen

Sports Risks

Prevalence HBV infects 0.4% of children and 0.8% of adults nationally, this is concentrated in endemic and super endemic communities. London schools and sports clubs will between two and ten times as infected as rural schools.

Costs UK sports children are often left unvaccinated for HBV due to cost effective issues. Cost has been a reason why at amateur boxer, martial artist, and wrestler and rugby levels infections are still common

Access Ignorance of risk and prevalence causes a large number of sports people to miss their protections. Many advisors, GP's and schools still forget to vaccinate. The biggest disaster is local education authorities wholesale avoiding plasters exactly when they are every bit as important as condoms. Whole schools are saying air is good for wounds, watching transmission routes in the playground and never testing the wounded.

Risk Assessment Transmission Routes That is the point with all this, just 3 pricks and you are infected. 10 rounds and you are infected. Unwashed boxing gloves and you are infected. Shared Rock holds and you are infected.

Deaths Liver cancer has killed a number of famous boxers

Fallacies. Many sports venues simply assume the infections never happen

Calls

Eric Abidal HBV positive footballer wonderful man won everything with Lionel Messi like the Euro Cup had liver cancer surgery at 30 and a transplant at 32, linked to web site offering information's, support and materials.

HBV positive Premiership Footballer Did not know enough about HBV

Boy 14 Sent to school boxing club got HBV same time School knew nothing about blood hygiene National sports bodies just as ignorant. Terrifyingly only the UK forgets to vaccinate its child and youth boxers

Boxer's wife. Hubby dying perhaps 4 weeks decompensating liver. Wife is in shock had never heard of HBV. Her favourite boxer Joe Frasier has just died also from liver cancer, hubby was also jaundiced in past during career. The "WHY" does no one talk about this was screaming here

About 100 Sports clubs and school teachers Explained that Premiership Blood Hygiene is the man on match of the day who at the sight of blood stops everything until the pitch, clothes and player are clean and plastered. That we have watched him since 1991 because since then we know blood spills to a wound in a contact sport is a 1 in 3 risk of HBV infection and yet not a playground in the UK offers this as basic mandatory care. Not a staff member in England has realised the children need this care on match of the day up to 20 times more due to their childish immunity, they can be wide open all day.

Chefs Builders Mechanics Glaziers

Gateway Wounds

Prevalence
HBV infects a surprisely large number of people who experience regular wounds. Over the years and many, many calls we have noted workers with wounds get HBV and HCV a lot more than others. These infections especially seem motored by two things, impact wounds and skin conditions.

Chefs Builders Mechanics Glaziers
On investigating wounds
Building Sites we noted every first aid kit was covered in blood.
Glaziers share blood on sharps quite often
Chefs work in a sort of a frenzy with constant wounds
Mechanics have often not used a plaster in their entire careers

Eczema, Bleach Cracks and Cutical Cuts

On investigating eczema and cutical cuts we found infections in

- Nurseries
- Schools
- Hospitals

Costs & Access
None of the above had training in blood hygiene, except the large constructors who had the filthiest first aid boxes. Ignorance of risk and prevalence causes a large number of workers to miss their protections. Many advisors, GP's, schools forget to vaccinate. None of the above would be advised of the risk. Crucially from Nursery onwards no one understands that a plaster each and every time is crucial, that blood to wound is a 100 times more infectious than sex with these viruses.

Risk Assessment Transmission Routes
That is the point with all this, just 3 pricks and you are infected.

Deaths Without risk and test awareness many will progress to cirrhosis
Fallacies. Many employers simply assume the infections never happen

STOP

34 million people have HIV
400 million have Hepatitis B
170 million have Hepatitis C

CAUTION

HIV, HBV and HCV Viruses
Can live in spilt blood and infect
Via contact with an open wound

USE

Gloves and scrubs
Fast plaster all wounds
Bleach kill the spill

BECAUSE

1 in 12 people in the world &
1 in 80 people in the UK
Bleed a blood virus now

"Premiership Blood Hygiene for every child and sport"
0800 206 1899

Blood Hygiene Precautions Factsheet

Blood has infected 2,000 million people with HBV; sex has only infected 34 million with HIV. It is that important to know your standard precautions when dealing with wounds and spilt blood.

We have become aware of the threat from water Bourne viruses e.g. cholera, and from air Bourne e.g. flu and sneezing on the underground and from sexual fluids e.g. HIV, but we are nationally falling short with blood borne e.g. viruses from transfusion or wound.

Firstly use plasters; with a blood virus it is always important to promptly plaster any flowing wound (a gateway for infection into your system). Remember one in 10 people on Earth now bleed blood viruses HBV, HCV, HIV, and use prompt plasters.

Secondly, watch where you bleed, it is necessary to think where spilt blood can live shared razors, shared DIY tools, and sharp milk teeth at school. Teach children, especially boys, that blood is in no way for display, a la Hollywood.

Thirdly, don't fight, in Australia, risk questioning found high numbers (most) of infected co-habiters have a history of domestic violence. Fighting is proven by the International Boxing Federation to transmit at a rate of every 10 rounds, so this risk needs to be taken very seriously. Also in the co-habiters of injectors, almost all of the infected reported needles stick injuries.

Fourthly, use only 10% Bleach and always wear gloves for cleaning spills. Only Bleach kills the virus out of the body via its heat. Other cleaning agents don't work. Hot, hot water can also be used if bleach is unavailable.

Post-exposure prevention
If you are not immunised and have been exposed to the virus, you should wash the wound area with hot water and be given an injection of antibodies called immunoglobulin within 48 hours. This may prevent infection from developing. Unfortunately we have had many calls wherein victims at high risk are repeatedly refused by many Accident and Emergency departments.

If Blood is the new Asbestos, Plasters are the new Condoms

A great deal of education is needed to get the protections enjoyed by wealthy footballers into our poorer, inner city school pitches. The Green Hepatitis Man stops any football match until all wounds are covered and blood removed and bleached. This has occurred since 1991, yet when a child raises their hand bleeding, all too often no one knows what to do. Basically there is no green man, no one who understands millions have got infected from such accidents.

Statistically, our children are 60 times more likely to touch infectious hepatitis blood than come across HIV in the course of their lives. Yet currently, in the UK you will be called alarming if you request milk teeth blood hygiene, even plasters at your local Primary School.

Children and workers with blood especially need training in the fact that if a HCV particle is equivalent in size to a marble, a syringe would be 75 miles high, i.e. it cannot be seen to be cleaned, it has to be killed with bleach. One drop of HCV blood has enough tiny viral particles to infect 100,000 people. Plus the enormous value of testing your liver status after and during years of service as a blood worker. With at least 40% of infections having no clear cause, unhygienic blood spill, is a major suspect.

In occupational settings, tattoo parlours, piercing venues, funeral and beautician parlours, barbers, cleaners, dental nurses, sports and other first aiders, emergency and security staff. In fact right across almost two million "blood workers" real education and training is needed. With schools we have developed a pack to teach this hygiene across the age ranges and within sports, biology and Public Health and Social Education, culminating in offering to 16 year olds enough information in how to keep their blood clean enough to donate.it at 18. Fully half of 18 teen year olds unknowingly are ineligible to donate as they have already run sexual or piercing or tattoo risks.

The simple facts about disease prevalence, globally 1 in 10 humans bleed a blood virus and the hepatitis death rate 1 in 10 undiagnosed viral infected die of cancer, have sparked blood hygiene globally. One of the worst questions when talking to school children, was being asked by an 8 year old who saw my plaster, "Why are you wearing that?" No child should wait until 8 to find an adult to answer because deadly viruses love an open wound. They had just admitted they all splashed blood everywhere like the movies for attention.

Chapter 4 Children - Hepatitis B & C Risks

PHE Surveillance notes 1 in 130 children has HBV in our hospitals

"Having imported a Devastating Child Pandemic into many of our homes and most of our schools, that is far more infectious than HIV, that is killing more than HIV in the developed world. We owe it to this generation and every generation infected as children to warn them."

Costs Another case of the closer to the super endemic community or blood HBV risk the less the awareness and budget for HBV vaccination or HBV and HCV testing is available. An Ethiopian family of 6 was quoted £1500 for HBV vaccinations, we often find ourselves recommending the UK Aid vaccinations already in Africa, Middle East & Asia.

Access To care is also frustrated by a complete lack of awareness of risk. Almost all Travel Advisors and GP's forget to vaccinate endemic community children. Many teaching staff have a zero plasters local education authority guidance and no background wherein blood hygiene is common. With some 30% of UK children born to endemic communities up to 4 million children are at frequent or very frequent risk of HBV infection.

Assessment Children present with serious risks until 11 and get infected the most during those years. Teething, Scratching, Biting, Falling over, Poking and even help Poohing are all normal development behaviors and therefore guaranteed risks here. Ignorance of risk and prevalence causes a large number of children to miss their protections. Time and again they touch blood and forget plasters.

Risk An 8.7% infection rate by 5 was noted among sub Saharan African children in a UK city in the Noughties, we repeatedly we note that
- Long stay children back to rural Afro Asia get infected
- Child Health Tourists get infected as overseas expect immunity
- FGM girls often all get infected
- Gap Year Students get infected
- Contact Sports and Climbers get infected

Globally boys are 80% more infected by 15 e.g. sports/wounds/fights.

Deaths Tragically 1% of our HBV & HCV children are end stage at 16.
Fallacies Pretending it is unnecessary to test our children and that HBV is different here to the rest of the world is politically correct spin instead of care.

Child Staff Calls

The worst thing about the numerous child carer calls is the shocked surprise children are infectious with HBV, a billion children have caught HBV so far, every time we test a Comprehensives worth of UK children in hospitals we find 18 children with HBV for the last 10 years. Shocked surprise is always total and it is just not where our child experts should be after 10 years with what is a highly infectious child virus.

- A School first aider infected by a pupil blood spill to wound, acute, cleared, but a year of misery.
- A Great Ormond St nursery carer infected via cutical cuts, chronic
- A Nursery carer caught HBV from a toddler blood spill
- School care taker caught chronic HBV from the blood spills
- 18, did St John first aid no vaccination her and partner HBV infected
- Teenage Assistant reported sharp milk teeth as a transmission route
- 16, asked to clean up blood, caught cHBV is a qualified doctor now.
- 17, asked to porter with hand eczema touched blood now acute HBV
- A Principal advised of 6 possible carriers admitted she already had caught HBV from a pupil

Child Institutional Infection Calls

- 19, had a kidney drain infected with HBV in London 2013
- 8, Manchester HBV infected during a transplant
- Another call concerned a disturbed HBV positive 17 teen year old in sheltered accommodation 5 of his carers and 2 other children had already experienced blood spills. We have had special needs related calls concerning hundreds possibly thousands in these situations

Child Tattoo/Beauty Calls

- 17, yellow, acute HBV from a tattoo, Morrison's Awareness Day
- 2 babies, 3 and 6 months HBV infected by a piercing gun, Norwich
- 17, botox party infection, chronic, 11 girls at party
- 18, Fresher's call – Chinese unwittingly transmitted her HBV to her first partner. Shared razors. Both quit their degrees. Both Chronic.

Child and Parent Calls

- 2, London pushchair, bright yellow acute met at Asda Awareness Day
- 14, Afghani boy never warned his blood is infectious, has lived with 60 people in foster families and shaves
- 4 girls one class all HBV infected west London school parent called. The point here is a phenomenon called classroom clustering. Globally every nation has noted groups of children at age 11 and 15 have HBV in the same class rather than spread across the year group evenly. This is highly indicative of onward spread in school, we have only confirmed a few of these but they present another urgent need to test and understand more this cancer causing virus in our schools.
- Parents often call when a school infection happens, no school co operates
- 5, nursery schoolgirl HBV infected at a Nurses Nursery, zero plasters.
- Many calls - For tens of thousands of children, there is no one with blood hygiene awareness
- 14, contracted HBV from the school boxing club,
- 8, infected boy who compass gamed with 14 children with the same needle,
- 14, in Gloucester shared injecting equipment, chronic HBV
- A baby infected when maternity forgot to stock the vaccination
- A teenager told by her GP father at 11 to hide her infection as she will be unmarriageable.
- 15, infected when his Granny from Pakistan borrowed his razor
- 9, caught chronic HBV borrowing parents toiletries
- A nurse's toddler denied Immuno globin at A and E after a needlestick
- 3 children HBV positive the dad was refused vaccinations as no risk
- 2 Chinese and 3 Somali under 12's taught first aid but not vaccinated Chinese Nurse mum utterly horrified

Child HBV Infection Travel Calls

- A 13 teen year old Ghanaian girl infected when sent overseas for female genital mutilation – sometimes all the girls at the cutting party are infected both overseas and more often lately here. Nigerian cutters are testing toward 25% HBV infected.
- 6 , went back to Malaysia mum forgot vaccination chronic infection
- 4, went back to Sierra Leone for a year chronic HBV infection
- 8, Pilipino sent back for visit and chronic HBV infected

Key HBV/HCV Risks for Children born overseas

Published medical reports below detail infection levels in young children, with HBV being far more infectious via blood spills its figures are worse. Do remember the snapshots below are small cohorts or individual schools. Orphandoctor.com screens whole schools for Hepatitis;

	HCV		HBV		
Spain	0.36%	Turkey	2.7%		
Pakistan	0.44%	Mexico	3.1% Girls	4.8% Boys	
Ukraine	1%	Crete	1.9%		
Brazil	4%	Nigeria	3.8% Girls	4.7% Boys	
Ghana	5.4%	Ghana	6%		
Cameroon	14.5%	Moldova	6%		

In the UK infection figures for schools have never been recorded and of course our NHS HCV infected children will be 18 or over by now. However massive unscreened migration from Pandemic areas will be, along with horizontal infections, in all our inner city schools. Imagining a low 0.02% infection level for HBV and a low 0.02% infection level for HCV could be a grave mistake for many multi cultural 2% HBV infected inner city UK schools.

We need the Hepatitis B and C atlases in schools along with the awareness the Pandemic is present with all its attendant blood hygiene rules and requirements taught in schools

Every child has a right to know blood is the most infectious body fluid
Most nations are doing a great deal more than we are to care for, and find these children. It is very important to realise most African and Asian countries have now progressed far with screening for and universally vaccinating these children, yet here most migrants from Pandemic areas are completely unaware how infected they are. With Mohammed being the most popular name in our schools, we could see the need for more testing and with HBV far, far more vaccinating. We could understand this child cohort is better diagnosed than going to University and early adulthood with all their perils, unaware of 20 years HCV or HBV infection.

Children Inspiring Calls

- 17 teen years old Almas rang shortly after her father died of liver cancer. Her mother, a Health Minister in Malawi, was horrified a man presenting with high risk and liver symptoms had not been tested over 30 years. Almas is studying healthcare with a focus on HBV border safety testing and HBV vaccination of its migrant populations at Canterbury
- Perhaps the best call was from a 15 teen year old girl, calm and quick to learn all about HBV. She developed the catch phrase for patient care for those diagnosed without liver problems "HBV? Great meds and great vaccs, no problem." She has been invaluable in designing wrap around family care and infectious to others with her managing plan, even her own mum has really benefited.
- Untouchable was diagnosed at 15 and avoided all human touch until 19, she had no idea millions of people with HBV get married. She helped develop the 7 point toddler/child/teen advice packs and pointed out being told you have an incurable 100 times more infectious cancer causing sex disease and asked if you do heroin, anal, oral or paid for sex in front of your mum and dad is a tough place to ask questions. She is studying healthcare communications at university now.

With the children most and the parents next and the GP's last we developed the following counselling and educations for HBV Kids & Families.

- Prognosis – how to live longer than most
- Relations and Children – how to fall in love and have children
- Vaccination - How to vaccinate and protect friends and loved ones
- Wisdom - Understanding their HBV, their Liver and their tests
- Premiership Blood Hygiene – Sterilise blood, wounds and razors etc.
- HBV Do's and Don'ts – Diet, Toxins, Attitudes
- Who to tell - People who love you enough to learn HBV & HCV

**"The simple truth is our migrant children are now the only ones left on Earth unprotected. They have been sacrificed for decades to the full horror of a preventable HBV Epidemic. We have a moral duty to diagnose them before even one more develops liver cancer.......
All of them, every last child, be it 50,000."**

Paul Desmond CEO www.hepbpositive.org.uk

Child concerning calls

We have had several calls regarding divorcees using HBV positive status as a reason to withhold access to a child, sometimes for nearly a year due to fumbling at the HBV vaccination 6 month course, then titre test at one year is the reasoning. Our feeling very much is if the courts agree to access this delay is bad for the child. In all our experience with diagnosed parents of unvaccinated children they observe rigorous precautions with their children when taught.

We have also had numerous calls from schools and parents advised that a HBV positive child is present. The problem is so little testing or vaccinating is done thereafter. The way the admission emerges helps everyone ignore the issue. The child tells his friend often after a bleed, the friend tells his mum and the mum tells the School Principal or us without naming the boy.
At this point the poor Principal searches for help, GP's will tell her "Don't worry just use condoms one day, Ofsted will say just use universal blood precautions. At this point some schools do a whiteboard session in the staff room and realise no one really knows

How to kill blood viruses in spills
The most common in school reasons for transmission
That a zero plaster policy is dangerously infectious
Someone always says that the HBV is 100 times more infectious than HIV and in the saliva after a search. Then they ring us this is actually a usual story from a flustered HR lady on the phone when they call. The concern is that this is common in our city schools now for 10 years and quite uniquely and carelessly we are the only nation on Earth without knowledge or a prevalence, going in and coming out, of what this child bug is doing in our schools.

Rituals
It is quite amazing how many different cultures have rituals that transmit viral Hepatitis B and C to children. We have had reports from

Ritual baby ear piercing by Hindus	Ritual blood brothering
Ritual cut throat shaving on Haj	Ritual scratch gang tattoo
Ritual Scarification African healer	Compass game
Ritual Circumcision male and female	Tooth touching games
Ritual Bleeding Islamic health	Unplastered wounds

It is an insane ritual in many schools that air is good for wounds

Poor Blood Hygiene Advice is given to HBV children

HBV positive children are not being told they have HBV until they are 14 or older. This means we get a lot of calls over the years from children of 15 or so, with mum and dad in the background so to speak. One of the biggest traumas is not their managed HBV infection, but all the people they love who they may have infected.

If these children are taught from a young age the important truth that blood and wounds are very infectious and as they grow older to strictly use plasters and blood hygiene a lot of this can be avoided. The explosions happen when stay over's have happened and other mums from Aunties and in laws start to worry and remember blood spills.

After the first 1,000 calls from people who acquired HBV during childhood or children at risk in 2011, we contacted some 50 countries health services for facts about child transmission, all reported HBV as caught mainly by children.

Ghana Most Hepatitis B (HBV) infections in sub-Saharan African infants and children are acquired through horizontal transmission from others

China The prevalence of HBV among children under 1 year of age is low but increases rapidly thereafter, reaching a peak among 5 to 9 year olds. Dr Yao

India Among family members, 19.4% were HBsAg positive and 37.6% positive for cleared HBV

Turkey It is concluded that generally the 7-11 year old period seems to be the most critical age in the horizontal transmission of HBV infection.

Japan The implementation of measures to prevent HBV horizontal infection is also essential, and the present system of selective vaccination should be expanded to universal vaccination.

Zambia Samples from 79 children and 80 adults, it was determined that new infections occurred during the five years of this study in at least 14 children (18%) (aged 4-17 years) and ten adults (12%)
Before HBV vaccination **Uganda, Morocco, USSR, Thailand** all noted 1 in 3 children catching HBV by age 15 in a WHO survey

Chapter 5 Travel - Hepatitis B & C Risks

Prevalence

Huge numbers travel overseas with no idea they are onward to a nation where 95% of people get HBV. On the national helpline each autumn we notice the holiday makers call with symptoms, no one seems aware that in half the world half the people catch HBV especially.

Costs

Another case of the closer to the super endemic community or blood risk the less the awareness and budget for HBV vaccination or for HBV and HCV testing. A family of 6 was quoted £1500 for HBV vaccinations, we often find ourselves recommending the UK Aid vaccinations already in Africa, Middle East & Asia on arrival at £5 each.

Access

Many Travel Advisors, GP's, Employers forget to vaccinate. They are also thousands suffering from vaccines being offered as 6 month courses with 2 weeks to departure. GP's must learn accelerated courses, this is critical.

Risk Assessment & Transmission Routes

With the WHO atlas of Infection still unused Ignorance of risk and prevalence causes a large number of travelers' to miss their protections. Repeatedly we note that

- Long stay children back to rural Afro Asia get infected from healthcare
- Health Tourists get infected as overseas expect immunity
- FGM girls often all get infected
- Holiday makers use casualty at lot and overseas expect immunity
- Sex Tourists to Bangkok and other destinations get infected
- Gap Year Students get infected
- Contact Sports and Climbers get infected
- There is a risk of death from initial HBV infection and travelers are often unable to pay for survival.

Deaths Tragically 2 stay in my mind a suicide and a lady too far from help.

Fallacies. Hepatitis B and C are rare and hard to get overseas.

Holiday & Travel Hepatitis B Helpline Calls

Many helpline caller reports show a national picture of ignorance.

1. "I went to Thailand and honestly not for a sexual escapade but after 2 months I met a lovely girl, who did not work in a bar and after meeting her parents, fell in love and planned to move there at some point. However on my return to the UK to earn more money for us both, I came down with HBV which has since become chronic. My girlfriend has since also tested positive as has her mother cHBV, father immune and brother cHBV. To say I am stunned is an understatement if a place has 70% HBV infection levels why are travellers not being told?"

2. "I am an Indian Asian and as is common went to India before my wedding to buy jewellery and my wedding sari. I also indulged in a lot of very economical beauty treatments, derma abrasion, manicures, pedicures, waxing, wedding henna markings and botox injections. On returning to the UK I got married and came down with HBV and my husband shortly thereafter. Basically the honeymoon period of my life was destroyed by HBV and now I am chronic and even children is something I am terrified of rather than look forward to, even sex is something I am frightened of now. Thank God my husband cleared the virus so at least I don't blame myself for that."
Wedding infections are also common as brides become most infectious 2 months after infection.

3. "We expected the holiday we would never forget, 9 weeks into our dream around the world journey my husband came down with fulminant HBV in Southern Italy, he was rushed to an isolation unit drifting into delirium going bright yellow. I googled that this could be the end of him and read sex is 100 times as infectious as HIV, so I was just sitting there watching the whites of his eyes going black imagining I would be keeling over soon. The costs emotionally and financially were crippling. Thank God I stumbled across Paul who emailed and took the calls and got some answers into my head. We feel that healthcare in Egypt where he had an accident or Cyprus where he had the stitches out and an injection was the source."

4. "I asked my GP for all the vaccinations and am flying in 3 days and have just heard of HBV being common in China where I am to teach English. Why on Earth did my GP not recommend a vaccination?"

5. "I plan a gap year in the third world as a Volunteer and am flying in 2 weeks, why do they not recommend the HBV vaccination?"

51

Holiday & Travel Hepatitis B Helpline Calls

We get many calls after Michael Palin shows from people HBV infected following his lead into third world street Dentist and Barber Chairs

6. "My husband went for 4 months work in Hong Kong and returned with HBV my GP led me to believe it was a sex disease so I kicked him out into the garage and he hung himself. I have since realised his extensive dentistry was probably the cause and am racked with guilt. Why wasn't he vaccinated? Why do GP's insist it is from sex and drug abuse?"

7. "I went for my bypass in Sri Lanka to avoid MRSA and have returned with HBV? Unfortunately the unit had no idea someone from the first world could be unvaccinated."

8. "I have been working as a Chef in Greece for a year and have contracted HBV, I have since discovered a workmate also has it, it is common here why does no one mention vaccination?"

9. "I caught HBV on holiday 6 years ago, why was I never referred? I had no idea it can kill people."

10. "I have just opened my results letter and found I have caught HBV on my holiday, I have another one for my husband I cannot open, am I going to die?"

11. "Hi, I am travelling tomorrow where do I get the HBV vaccination?"

12. "I returned from aid work in the Sudan to discover I had contracted HBV, why was I not vaccinated by my GP?"

13. "I often do business in China and seem to have caught HBV there, why was I not vaccinated?"

14. "I have spent 8 months in Thailand and have come back with HBV."

15. "I have had tetanus shot for a cut in the Philippines and come back with HBV."

16. "I got HBV having my baby in Pakistan from the clinic and gave it to my hubby, both chronic!"

17. Team of doctors sent back from China as forgot HBV vaccination
18. Team of doctors sent back from Serbia as forgot HBV vaccination

19. "I went to Sierra Leone, little realising that the reason was for my female circumcision, on my return I found I was going yellow at school and diagnosed with HBV. It is only now I am at University and out of home I am searching for answers to all this."

20. "I am very confused I asked my GP for a HBV vaccination and he said he would not give me one on the NHS, I pleaded can I pay, he then said there is no risk in India and he is not vaccinated. My father has died of HBV in India, is it so odd to demand a vaccination?"

21. "I am flying to Turkey for a job in 2 weeks I just cannot find a doctor, a chemist anyone anywhere in the UK to vaccinate me for HBV, why?"

22. "I took the family to see relatives in Nigeria for 2 months, on returning our two boys have come down with HBV. We have since learnt my family had many HBV carriers and we stayed with them. Why does no one talk about this problem, we had so many vaccinations but not the ones we needed."

23. "I am a medical intern and was due to work in a Indian hospital during my break from studies but have just been advised by them that my HBV vaccination is inadequate, I told my GP my intention 6 months ago, why has he left it until 2 weeks before I fly to start vaccinating?"

24. "My father is dying of HBV liver cancer in Canada, the Canadian visa people are advising a HBV vaccination and my GP has advised he cannot vaccinate me as it takes 6 months, help." We got a accelerated course for this lady and she flew after shot 2 in 7 days.

25. "I am HBV positive and pregnant and onward to Dubai." We pointed out that people who declare HBV have been interned and returned

26. "I asked my doctor for HBV vaccination as I am onward to China for a year and had 2 injections 9 years ago, he offered a booster injection?" Wrong a repeat course and a titre test is needed.

27. I used a used razor left on a sink at cologne airport I am HBV positive

28. I went to Malta as I have for years and without realising must have caught HBV from the barbers there, I love being groomed on my holidays, massages shaves etc. On return I was diagnosed with leukaemia about 3 months later I started the treatment and promptly went into a coma with a ALTs score of 2500. It emerged I had HBV and this reaction needed an air ambulance to a special Intensive Care unit and I survived. I was amazed when Paul told me that this is often happening as we do not always check for HBV with leukaemia patients. Our concern is 1.6% nationally and 2% of London patients are doing this and we are getting too many calls from coma cases, testing all leukaemia patients is surely needed and cost effective now as elsewhere.

29. We travelled to India and have just discovered our nanny of 2 months is HBV positive the baby is teething, we are horrified, why is there no warnings? We all had a strongly recommended flu jab in September and travelled in October but no one mentioned HBV. Flu is for a week HBV is for life!

The need for HBV vaccination among travelling migrant children

The US which vaccinates all newborns since 1993, now has 30 times less childhood infections than the UK, as a result. Currently without protection 10% of our HBV Positive population are children which equates to 50,000 of our children being infected over the last two decades.

With so many of our children moving unvaccinated within high prevalence countries and communities we need to diagnose and protect all our children fast. All migrants should be able to learn if their homelands recommend HBV child vaccinations before travelling. Schools need far more anonymous notification of returning HBV infections, when making test and vaccination decisions for your families remember

- HBV is incurable for up to 90% of children who catch it
- UK Child Paediatric Wards 2007-2015 have registered 1 in 140 children have HBV, a growing 0.8% prevalence.
- HBV globally kills more often than Malaria
- UK ethnic children were 8.7% HBV infected by 5 in a NHS Report
- We have had endless calls where GP's have denied a risk

Chapter 6 Migration Risks for Hepatitis B (Child Hepatitis)

Many millions of migrants have now been denied or cannot access their recommended HBV safety testing or vaccinations.

During the largest UK immigration boom in our history, we have mass imported 3% HBV positive people from nations that are just rolling out their own programmes for vaccinating and screening for Hepatitis B. We have done this without testing, warning or vaccinating any of these HBV endemic new citizens, as a result UK liver disease and deaths have boomed.

All 15 million migrants to the UK and their descendants are generally unable to access test warnings regarding their 3% infection levels and just as important, child vaccinations. As our predicted tripling of liver disease happens to them, all are in dire need of the standard health care usually deployed to endemic populations. Namely universal vaccination and safety testing.

High Risk Groups for Hepatitis B

Risk Group	UK Numbers at risk needing testing
Migrants from countries with high prevalence and UK born dependants	**13m**
Unvaccinated UK Children in our endemic communities & schools	**3m**
Families and household contacts of persons infected with HBV	**2m**
Workers who deal with blood Security, Sports, Cleaners	**2m**
Healthcare workers, especially First aiders and Carers	**1m**
People who have unsafe sex with many partners	**4m**
People who have been imprisoned or sectioned	**0.9m**
People who have ever injected or regularly snorted street drugs	**0.7m**
Men who have sex with men	**0.5m**
Female Genital Mutilation Survivors	**0.2m**

People who have received overseas reusable syringe injections
People who have operations in Africa, Asia, S America and East EU
People who had blood products e.g. c-sections, heamophiliacs
People who have had Heamodialysis

Patients with liver cirrhosis or fibrosis
Patients with Liver or Bile Duct Cancers
Patients with HIV
Patients with elevated liver enzymes and/or symptoms of hepatitis
Patients on immune suppressants or chemotherapy

Newborns of HBV infected mothers
People with tattoo's and piercings from unhygienic parlours

The European Liver Patients Association and
The European Association for the Study of the Liver and
The Hepatitis B Trust
Recommend safety testing for all those above

1 in 4 humans innocently catch Hepatitis B (HBV)
Testing your risk is nothing to be ashamed of

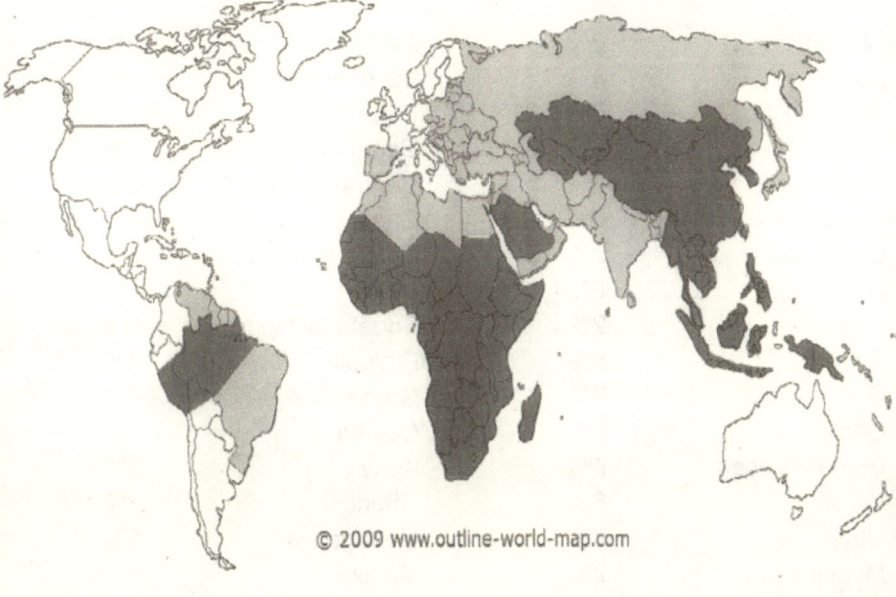

© 2009 www.outline-world-map.com

Under 2% | 2% | 7%

Hepatitis B is a virus that over 30 years can "silently" cause cirrhosis and cancer; a million people die each year worldwide due to late diagnosis. Millions of UK citizens are at risk. Hepatitis B infects without symptoms and most catch it as children from:

- Childhood Infection in any of the coloured areas above
- Re-used medical syringes in the coloured areas above
- Spilt blood to an unplastered wound when unvaccinated
- A period of jaundice (going yellow)
- HBV can also be transmitted by unprotected sex and
- The Injecting of illegal drugs (even once)

If you run any of the above risks or are planning a trip to an endemic area (shaded on the map) ask your GP about a Hepatitis B Safety Test and Vaccination. Remember Hepatitis B patients often have no symptoms until real damage has been done so knowing your status can help you safeguard your future.

0800 206 1899   Remember to ask your GP

Percentage of Population with Hepatitis B

Africa   6.75%

Algeria	2%	Angola	8%
Benin	8%	Botswana	8%
Burkina Faso	8%	Burundi	8%
Cameroon	8%	Canary islands	2%
Cape Verdi	2%	Central African Rep	8%
Ceuta	8%	Chad	8%
Comoros	2%	Cote d Ivorie	8%
DR Congo	8%	Djibouti	8%
Egypt	2%	Equatorial Guinea	8%
Eritrea	8%	Ethiopia	8%
Gabon	8%	Gambia	8%
Ghana	9%	Guinea	8%
Guinea-Bissau	8%	Kenya	9%
Lesotho	8%	Liberia	8%
Libya	2%	Madagascar	8%
Madeira	2%	Malawi	8%
Mali	8%	Mauritania	8%
Mauritius	2%	Mayotte	8%
Melilla	8%	Morocco	2%
Mozambique	8%	Namibia	8%
Niger	8%	Nigeria	14%
R Congo	8%	Reunion	2%
Rwanda	8%	Senegal	8%
Seychelles	2%	Sierra Leone	8%
Somalia	9%	South Africa	6.85%
Sudan	8%	Swaziland	8%
Tanzania	8%	Togo	8%
Tunisia	2%	Uganda	9%
Western Sahara	8%	Zambia	8%
Zimbabwe	8%		

HBV Population Percentages by Nation

Africa   6.75%

Nearly all of Africa suffered 50 to 80% rates of HBV infection due to the use of un sterile vaccine guns, reused syringes, Female Genital Mutilation and childhood horizontal transmissions. From the 1950's up until the rolling out of national newborn vaccinations across the Noughties, infections were up to 95%, Somalia and South Sudan were the last countries to introduce vaccinations in 2013.

From a general continental view, all persons from Africa would be recommended for rapid Hepatitis B and C screening and HBV vaccination, especially their children would need HBV vaccination as children are up to 20 times more likely to become lastingly HBV infected if they catch it.

One in fifty under five children a year was found to be catching HBV in a Liverpool African community in 2003, so the need for African parents to protect their children in the UK is huge.

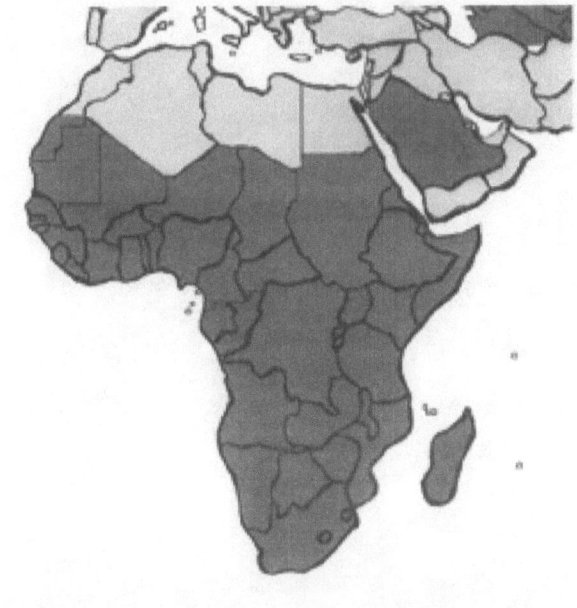

Under 2%   2 %   7%

Percentage of Population with Hepatitis B

Asia	7.5%	Middle East	6.75%
Afghanistan	8%	Armenia	8%
Azerbaijan	8%	Bahrain	2%
Bangladesh	4.5%	Bhutan	2%
Cambodia	8%	China	8.6%
Cyprus	4.5%	Fiji	8%
Georgia	8%	India	3.5%
Indonesia	8%	Iran	4.5%
Iraq	8%	Israel	2%
Japan	2%	Jordan	2%
Kazakhstan	8%	Kuwait	2%
Kyrgyzstan	8%	Laos	8%
Lebanon	2%	Malaysia	8%
Maldives	2%	Mongolia	8%
Myanmar	8%	Nepal	2%
North Korea	8%	Oman	8%
Pakistan	3.3%	Palau	8%
Philippines	10%	Qatar	2%
Russia	2%	Saudi Arabia	8%
Singapore	8%	South Korea	8%
Sri Lanka	4.5%	Syria	2%
Tajikistan	8%,	Thailand	8%
Turkey	4.2%	Turkmenistan	8%
United Arab Emirates	2%	Uzbekistan	8%
Vietnam	8%	Yemen	8%

"Know Your Hepatitis B & C Risks, and get them tested."

HBV Population Percentages by Nation

Asia 7.5% Middle East 6.75%

Nearly all of Asia suffered 30 to 80% rates of HBV infection due to the use of un sterile vaccine guns, reused health syringes and childhood horizontal transmissions. From the 1950's up until the rolling out of national newborn vaccinations campaigns, the majority of people in these nations caught HBV. Mercifully HBV vaccinations for newborns became complete in Asia in 2006, the last countries after 2000 were India, Afghanistan and Japan.

From a general continental view, all persons from Asia would be recommended for rapid Hepatitis B and C screening and HBV vaccination, especially their children would need HBV vaccination as children are up to 20 times more likely to become lastingly HBV infected if they catch it. On testing UK South Asians (Indian Sub continent) in 2003, it was noted that 9% of infections were in the under 15 group. This indicates onward spread amongst children is half of total infections, so the need for Asian parents to protect their children in the UK is as huge as in their nations of origin.

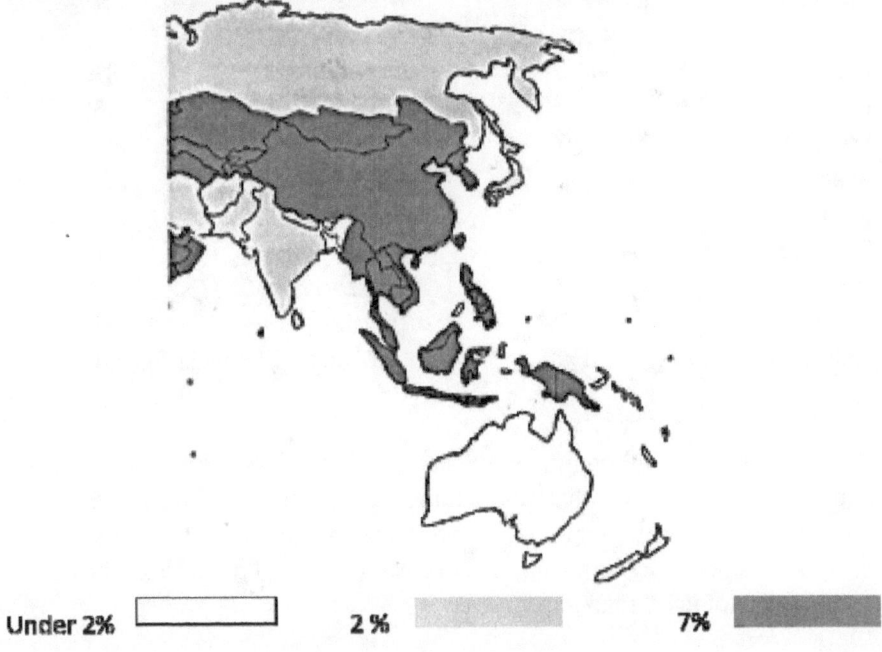

Under 2%　　　　　2 %　　　　　7%

Percentage of Population with Hepatitis B

Europe   1%

Albania	8%	Andorra	2%
Armenia	8%	Austria	.3%
Azerbaijan	8%	Belarus	2%
Belgium	.3%	Bosnia & Herzegovina	2%
Bulgaria	5%	Croatia	2%
Cyprus	4.5%	Czech Republic	.3%
Denmark	.3%	Estonia	2%
Finland	.3%	France	.3%
Georgia	8%	Germany	.5%
Greece	2%	Hungary	2%
Iceland	.3%	Ireland	.5%
Italy	2.4%	Kosovo	2%
Latvia	2%	Liechtenstein	.3%
Lithuania	2%	Luxembourg	.3%
Macedonia	2%	Malta	2%
Moldova	8%	Monaco	.3%
Montenegro	2%	Netherlands	.3%
Norway	.3%	Poland	1.5%
Portugal	.3%	Romania	2%
Russia	2%	San Marino	2%
Serbia	2%	Slovakia	2%
Slovenia	2%	Spain	2%
Sweden	.3%	Switzerland	.3%
Turkey	4.2%	Ukraine	2%
United Kingdom	1%	Vatican City (Holy See)	2.4%

Correction Note – On the map opposite we have marked Bulgaria, Moldova and Albania as more highly HBV infected than on the map on page 57. We have done this because after taking so many helpline calls from these nationalities and also contacting their health professionals we feel they are rather more infected than 2%.

HBV Population Percentages by Nation

Europe has a visible divide where injection gun use in the former soviet states caused them 2% plus HBV national levels, there is also a north south divide wherein Spain, Greece and Italy also have 2% levels. From the 1950's up until the rolling out of national newborn vaccinations campaigns 10-30% of these nations caught HBV. Throughout the EU mainland vaccinating newborns was complete by 2000; however the UK instead of testing or vaccinating has become the only place on Earth with rapidly increasing levels of child infection being reported by PHE Surveillance.

From a general continental view, all persons from Eastern and Southern Europe would be recommended for rapid Hepatitis B and C screening and HBV vaccination, especially their children would need HBV vaccination as children are up to 20 times more likely to become lastingly HBV infected if they catch it. The National HBV Helpline has taken huge numbers of calls from eastern and southern EU parents astonished that we do not use this crucial vaccination to protect their at risk children. Many were doctors or health professionals; they were the hardest calls as they knew clearly the dangers best

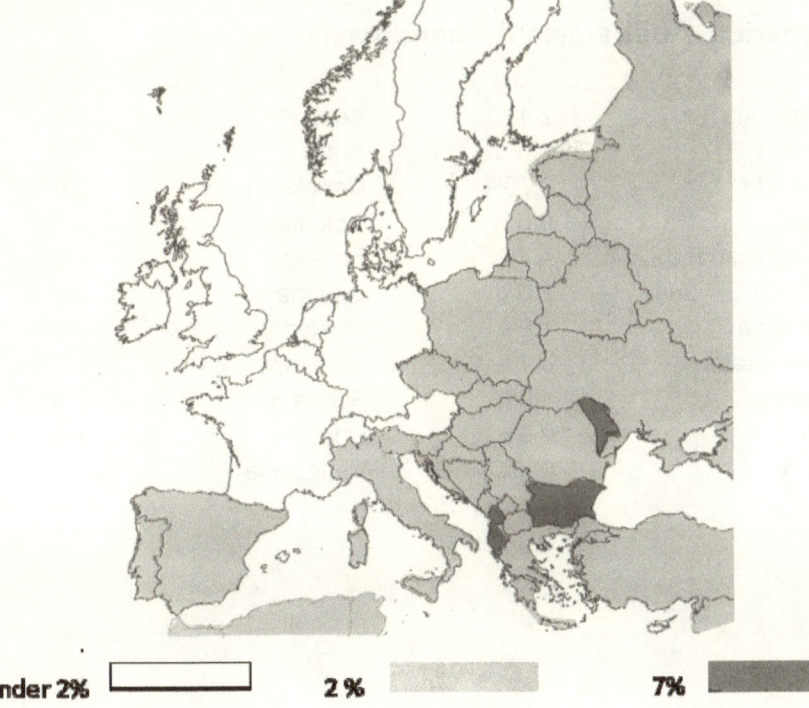

Under 2%   2 %   7%

HBV Population Percentages by Nation
America, Australasia & Scandinavia

Across the Americas and Australasia indigenous peoples namely the Inuit, Amazonian and Aboriginal citizens have super endemic levels of infection.

Latin Nations south of Mexico are endemic for HBV, and are also recommended for safety HBV testing and HBV vaccinations.

Western EU, North American & Australasian nations all note 3% of migrants have HBV on arrival and diagnose and care for them and their families on arrival and vaccinate their children as a precaution also.

However in the UK, in 2014 the Minister for Public Health refuses to believe any migrants here have HBV or discuss our PHE figures that adults now test 1.6% HBV infected nationally and ethnic groups at up to 10% regionally.

Percentage of Population with Hepatitis B

America, Australasia & Scandinavia

Argentina	2.1%	Australia	0.9%
Bolivia	1.0%	Brazil	5.9%
Canada	0.75%	Caribbean	0.9%
Chile	0.6%	Columbia	1.0%
Dominican Republic	4.4%	Ecuador	3.0%
French Guyana	2.0%	Guyana	2.0%
Jamaica	1.9%	Mexico	1.4%
New Zealand	0.7%	Paraguay	1.0%
Peru	4.0%	Surinam	2.0%
UK	0.8%	Uruguay	1.0%
USA	0.3%	Venezuela	3.2%

Chapter 7
Migration Risks for Hepatitis C (Healthcare Hepatitis)

Many millions of migrants have been denied or cannot access their recommended healthcare HCV risk facts or safety testing.

During the largest UK immigration boom in our history, and during a period when all the worlds borders that test note 1.5% of migrants have HCV. Our migrants have arrived just as their home nations are rolling out their own programmes for screening for healthcare Hepatitis C. We have not tested or warned any of the 12 million migrants of their homelands recommendations.

Nearly all UK migrants and their dependents are unable to access HCV test warnings regarding their 1.5% infection levels or the excellent cures now available. As our predicted tripling of liver disease happens to them, all are in dire need of the standard health care usually deployed to endemic populations, namely HBV universal vaccination and HCV safety testing and treatment.

The scale of overseas healthcare infections is dramatic, many nations used vaccine guns, and Egypt infected 15% of its population with just one vaccine gun campaign in 1979. One in forty humans contracted HCV from their health services, the WHO outbreak atlas of the disaster is still needed by our GP's and hospitals. (see next page)

It is quite incredible 250 million people catch HCV from their healthcare providers and our UK media is too censored to even tell our doctors about it.

High Risk Groups for Hepatitis C

Risk Group	UK Numbers at risk Needing testing

In Africa, Asia, Sth America and Eastern and Southern Europe

• People who have had overseas healthcare reusable injections	**10m**
• People who have had overseas operations	**0.5m**

In the UK and EU before 1992

• People who had operations	**1m**
• People who had transfusions or transplants	**1m**
• People who had blood products e.g. c-sections, heamophiliacs	**0.5m**

• Healthcare workers and all workers who deal with blood	**2m**
• People who have ever injected or snorted street drugs	**0.8m**
• Persons with elevated liver enzymes or symptoms of hepatitis	**0.5m**
• Female Genital Mutilation Survivors	**0.2m**
• Patients with liver cirrhosis or fibrosis	
• People who have been imprisoned or sectioned	
• People who have had Heamodialysis	
• People with HIV	
• People with tattoo's and piercings from unhygienic parlours	
• Children of HCV infected mothers	

The European Liver Patients Association and

The European Association for the Study of the Liver and

The Hepatitis B Trust

Recommend safety testing for all those above

200 Million Patients caught Hepatitis C (HCV)
Testing your risk is nothing to be ashamed of

HCV is a virus that over 20 years can silently cause cirrhosis, citizens who have run overseas healthcare or NHS risks are recommended for testing

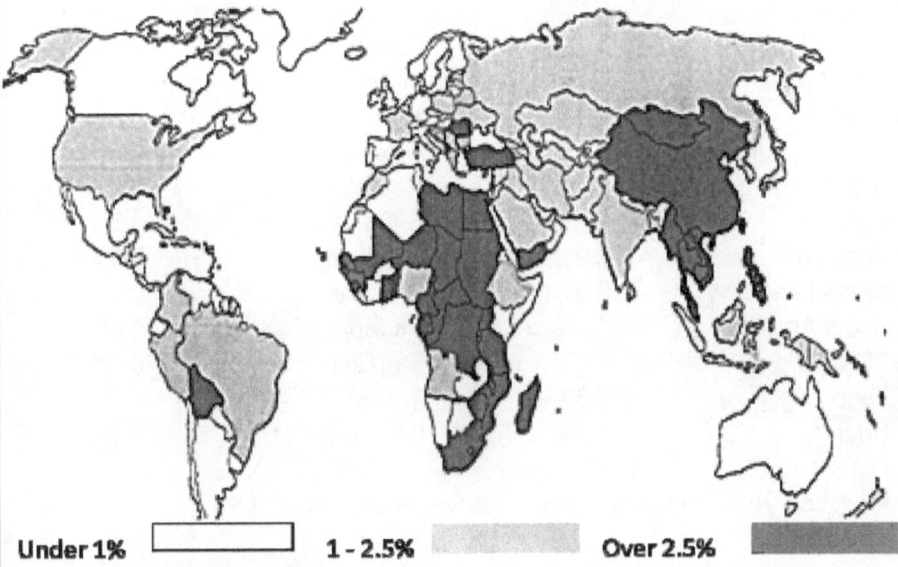

Under 1% 1 - 2.5% Over 2.5%

Patients can get Hepatitis C from

NHS Surgery or Dialysis before 1992
NHS C-section from before 1994
NHS Transfusions or blood products before 1993
Until 2000 these healthcare risks were usually higher overseas
Use the map above to understand your risk

Most Hepatitis C patients have no symptoms until damage has been done. So if you have run any of the above healthcare risks or have ever injected street drugs ask about a Hepatitis C safety test.

0800 206 1899   Remember to ask your GP

Africa - Percentage of Population with Hepatitis C

Algeria	0.2%	Angola	1.0%
Benin	1.5%	Burundi	11.1%
Cameroon	12.5%	Central African Rep.	4.5%
Chad	4.8%	Congo (Dem. Rep.)	6.4%
Egypt	18.1%	Ethiopia	2.0%
Gabon	6.5%	Ghana	2.8%
Guinea	10.7%	Kenya	0.9%
Madagascar	3.3%	Mauritania	1.1%
Mauritius	2.1%	Morocco	1.1%
Mozambique	2.1%	Niger	2.5%
Nigeria	1.4%	Reunion Island	0.8%
Rwanda	1.7%	Saudi Arabia	1.8%
Senegal	2.9%	Seychelles	0.8%
Sierra Leone	2.0%	Somalia	0.9%
South Africa	1.7%	Sudan	3.2%
Swaziland	1.5%	Tanzania	0.7%
Togo	3.3%	Tunisia	0.7%
Uganda	1.2%	Zimbabwe	7.7%

Morocco 2007 The HCV prevalence was estimated at **1.93%**.

Nigeria 2005 A prevalence of **2.9%** was observed in this study rising to (8.1%) of adults aged between 26 and 33 among blood donors

Pregnant Nigerian women 2005 **9.2%** were positive and 1.1% of the babies.

Saudi Arabia - HCV Levels
HCV seroprevalence in Saudi blood donors is estimated to be **3.5%,**

Somalia - HCV infection in chronic liver disease
HCV was studied in 110 patients with chronic liver diseases, in 309 healthy adults and in 287 children with diseases other than hepatitis. HCV was present in three healthy adults **0.97%.**

Uganda Prevalence of Hepatitis C virus 2006
We investigated 2592 plasma specimens collected consecutively from blood donors in central Uganda in 1999. 107 **4.1%** specimens were HCV.

Africa - Hepatitis C Population percentages by nation

"The Innocence of being operated on or trusting an inoculation accompanies Africa and the third world's Hepatitis B & C Pandemics not Stigma"

Madam Jehan Al Sadat.
President of the Egyptian Blood Bank

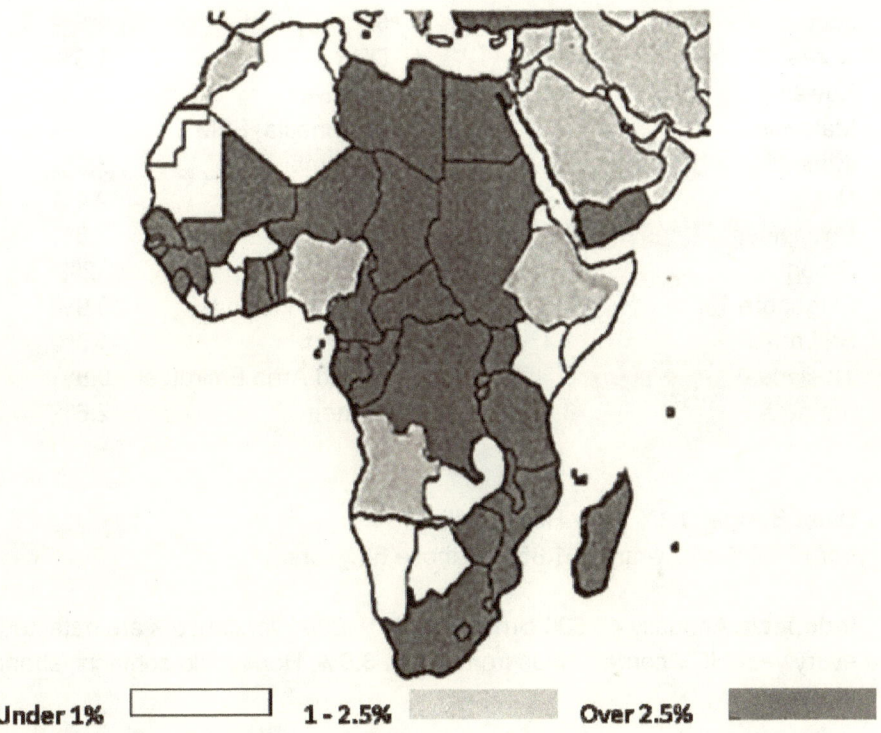

Under 1%   1 - 2.5%   Over 2.5%

Published African Medical Reports

Ethiopia - A Survey of Hepatitis C Virus HCV was measured in 1,580 Ethiopian subjects representing urban and rural populations. The HCV prevalence was **2%**. In Ethiopia, syringes and needles may be contaminated,

Egypt - Ignorance blamed for prevalence of Hepatitis C 2008. About **10%** have the virus. The high rate has resulted from the re use of syringes.

Ghana - Prevalence of HCV in Blood Donors 2002 The seroprevalence of HCV infection among blood donors was confirmed to be **0.9%**

Percentage of Population with Hepatitis C

Bangladesh	2.4%	Bhutan	1.3%
Cambodia	4.%	China	3%
Hong Kong	0.5%	India	1.8%
Indonesia	2.1%	Iraq	0.5%
Israel	0.4%	Japan	2.3%
Jordan	2.1%	Kiribati	4.8%
Korea, South	1.7%	DPR Korea	1.6%
Kuwait	3.3%	Maldives	1.8%
Malaysia	3%	Micronesia, FSM	1.5%
Mongolia	10.7%	Myanmar	3.9%
Nepal	0.9%	Pakistan	2.4%
Philippines	3.6%	Qatar	2.8%
Oman	0.9%	Russia	2%
Singapore	0.5%	Solomon Islands	0.9%
Sri Lanka	1.4%	Taiwan	1.6%
Thailand	5.6%	United Arab Emirates	0.8%
Vietnam	6.1%	Yemen	2.6%

West Bengal 0.8% were HCV positive
from 0.31% <10 years to 1.85% in those 60 years.

Indonesia Annually 45,000 cirrhosis and 18,000 liver cancers are detected
every year HCV carrier status from **2.1 to 3.9%.** Household contacts, sharing
(razors)

Korea HCV prevalence **1.6%,** 30.5% of cirrhosis of liver, 30% in Liver Cancer.

Maldives project HCV positivity in the population of Maldives as **1.8%.**

Myanmar
During 1997-98, of 1018 blood donors, 103(**10.1%**) were reactive for HCV

Nepal The blood donors were **1.8%** in 1996.

Sri Lanka HCV in Sri Lanka is reported to be **1.4%**

Thailand The population has HCV infection ranging between **0.5 and 5.6%**

Asia & Middle East HCV Population Percentages by Nation

"Hepatitis B and C have silently infected 2-7% of Asia's populations, if you have lived here and run a HBV or HCV risk. Get Tested"

Imran Khan Cricketer and Politician

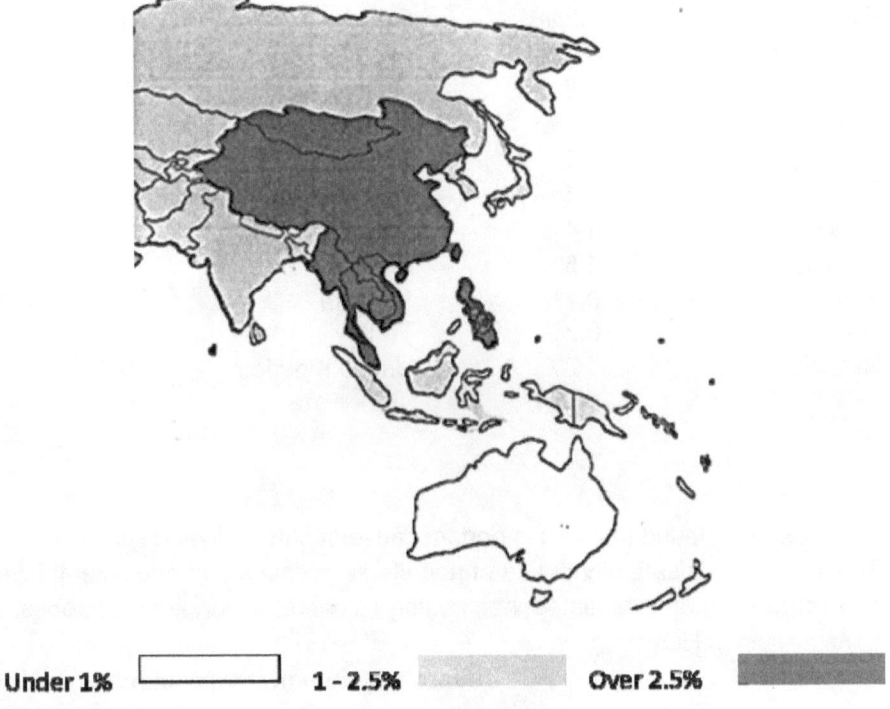

Under 1%　　　　　1 - 2.5%　　　　　Over 2.5%

Extracts from Published Asian Medical Reports

Bangladesh 2.4% HCV positivity in professional blood donors has been demonstrated; 45.3% of the primary hepatocellular carcinoma cases were HCV positive

Bhutan The HCV prevalence in the general population of Bhutan is **1.3%**

India It is estimated that there are 12.5 million HCV carriers **1%** in our country,
Pakistan
2006 sero-prevalence was **5% for HCV** and **2.5 % for HBV**. Risks from injections. HBV vaccine for newborns regardless of maternal HBV is needed.

Percentage of Population with Hepatitis C

Austria	0.2%	Belarus	1.4%
Belgium	0.9%	Bulgaria	1.1%
Croatia	1.4%	Cyprus	0.7%
Czechoslovakia	0.2%	Denmark	0.2%
Finland	0.2%	France	1.1%
Germany	0.1%	Greece	1.5%
Hungary	0.9%	Iceland	0.1%
Ireland	0.1%	Italy	0.5%
Luxembourg	0.5%	Moldova	4.9%
Netherlands	0.1%	Norway	0.1%
Poland	1.4%	Portugal	0.5%
Romania	4.5%	Slovakia	0.4%
Spain	0.7%	Sweden	0.3%
Switzerland	0.2%	Turkey	1.5%
Ukraine	1.2%	United Kingdom	0.7%

HCV has been found to be an important cause of chronic liver diseases. Transfusion of unsafe blood, use of non-sterile syringes and equipment, inject able drug use and repeated haemodialysis were major known modes of transmission of HCV.

Dr Sudarshan Kumari, Regional Adviser, WHO

Europe - Hepatitis C Population percentages by nation

"The European Union has a crucial role in identifying best practice with regard to Hepatitis B & C screening. One in 50 Europeans has HBV or HCV."

Stephen Hughes, Public Safety, European Parliament

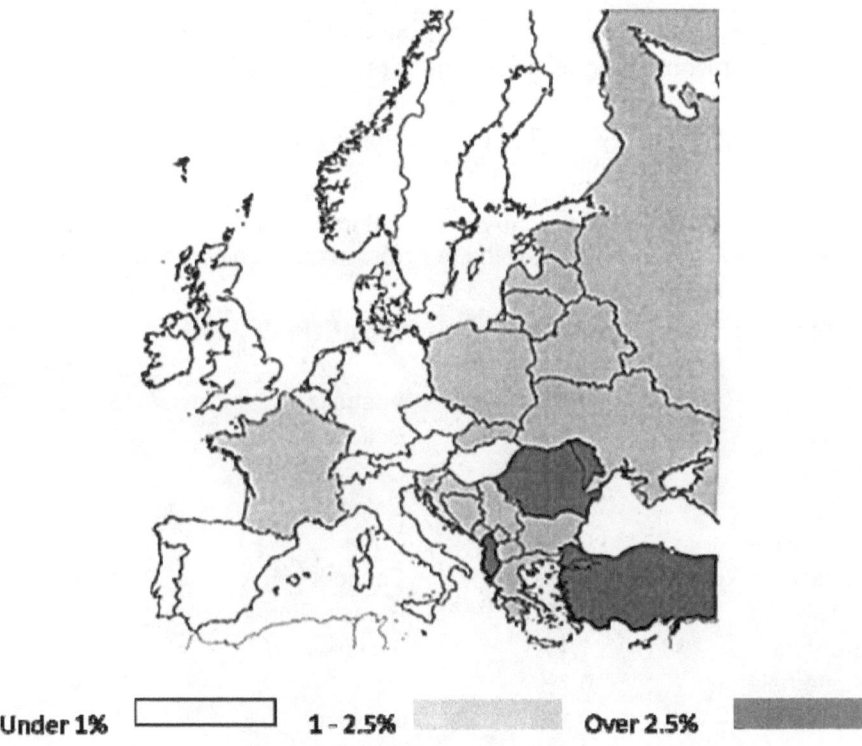

Under 1%   1 - 2.5%   Over 2.5%

Major EU Risk Factors for Hepatitis C
- Had a EU major surgery or transfusion or blood products before1992
- Had EU Dialysis or Organs
- Shared equipment for injecting drugs
- Had injection or surgical transfusion in high prevalence countries
- Had needle stick injuries (emergency and health workers)

Majority of Europeans with Hepatitis C remain undiagnosed
"It is alarming that in the twenty-first century there are European countries where up to 90% of people with HBV & HCV may not know they are infected",

Nadine Piorkowsky, President, European Liver Patients Association

HCV Population Percentages by Nation

America, Australasia & Scandinavia

Key Risks include

- Healthcare Injections and Inoculations before 1992
- Operations using blood or organs or dialysis before 1992
- Street Injecting and unsterile tattoos
- In Canada, Brazil and Australia, the Inuit, Amazonian tribal and Aborigine all have 4% levels of HCV

The US admit 240,000 infections per annum from Healthcare dropping to 20,000 from IDU's after 1993, with the screening of all blood and products.

Percentage of Population with Hepatitis C

Argentina	0.6%	Australia	0.3%
Belize	0.1%	Bolivia	11.2%
Brazil	2.6%	Canada	0.1%
Chile	0.9%	Colombia	1.0%
Costa Rica	0.3%	Cuba	0.8%
Dominican Republic	2.4%	Ecuador	0.7%
El Salvador	0.2%	French Guiana	1.5%
Grenada	1.1%	Guadeloupe	0.8%
Guatemala	0.7%	Haiti	2.0%
Honduras	0.1%	Jamaica	0.3%
Mexico	0.7%	New Zealand	0.3%
Nicaragua	0.6%	Paraguay	0.3%
Peru	1.6%	Puerto Rico	1.9%
Suriname	5.5%	Trinidad and Tobago	4.9%
United States	1.8%	Venezuela	0.9%

"It is estimated that approximately 250 million persons worldwide and over 5 million Americans have Hepatitis C from healthcare or drug abuse, and that the majority are unaware of their exposure, baby boomer and migrant testing is crucial care."

Mr Chris Kennedy Lawford is an eminent US Addiction Author and a National US HCV Spokesperson, along with being a Hollywood actor and nephew of the former President.

Chapter 8 Mother to baby HBV & HCV Risks

NHS Maternity Units and Midwives are excellent at avoiding mother to baby infections. Having met hundreds at various conferences, every mum with HBV or HCV needs to know straight away that they are in good hands and

Baby will be fine

One aspect of running the Hepatitis Helpline is the amazing army of HBV Moms that ring, nearly all these ladies are in profound shock as they have never had a symptom and never run a risk they knew about. At 3 months pregnant, usually with their first born, hardly one has a clue about HBV, it is really important to get across straight away, **you and your baby will be fine**

In the 10 years since we started the helpline and following hundreds of mums, only one baby has got infected and that was because a rural clinic had no stock of vaccine. But this means nearly 50,000 births since 2002 and only one report. Among the hundreds of babies and mums we have watched get through things, it is the 7 point counselling for families with diagnosis that works best.

- Prognosis – how to live longer than most

This is crucial with baby on the way, easy to do with an early diagnosis and a liver good life approach.

- Relations and Children – how to fall in love and have children

Having the vaccination schedule handy, being able to get an accelerated course over 21 days really empowers patients to ask partners to get protected and try dating. Knowing babies are all safe now also stops couples sterilising themselves after one baby.

- Vaccination - How to vaccinate and protect friends and loved ones

It is very important to be able to access vaccinations and GP's will often fail so knowing Lloyds Pharmacy offers the vaccine is good for all the people they refuse like uncles and lodgers and children to HBV dads

- Wisdom - Understanding HBV, the Liver and their tests

Mums need to know they are fine and the blood tests need to be explained and one by one prove it. It is lack of a book on HBV that is the problem, not their desire to learn.

- Premiership Blood Hygiene – Sterilise blood, wounds and razors etc.

Every mum and hepatitis patient really benefits from this, knowing basic nurse hygiene with blood. We have a nursery rhyme we use with tots that helps. Use gloves and scrubs, Plaster the disaster, And Bleach kill the spill. Confidence flows from knowing this, mums whose babies are safe often create hygiene in nurseries and schools for the other children who are still susceptible to infection.

- HBV Do's and Don'ts – Diet, Toxins, Attitudes

A HBV mums first shop, avoiding fried and fatty foods going lean meats etc is a joy to behold, the list is on page 127.

- Who to tell - People who love you enough to learn HBV or HCV

Mums are in the front line of testing and caring for their parents and siblings. It is often a benefit to mums to diagnose and get into care other uncles and cousins etc.

The point here is 5000 HBV mums are the vast bulk of our HBV patients and they have a right to the quality printed facts above so they can manage HBV calmly and quickly and get on with having a baby. Far too many become deeply depressed or anxious needing tranquilisers, some even have terminations or relationship issues, all for want of information. There is little joy in being excellent at avoiding mum to baby infections, if the patient is cringing in terror for 9 months to find out. If you could hear the mums cry down the phone when they know their baby is finally safely vaccinated, you would understand why we need the above counselling fast for everyone's health. This one page is so important, it's a chapter and I bet lots of Just Diagnosed mums will turn to this page first.

HBV Dads, outnumber mums by two to one.

No word about HBV mums should be said without mentioning the 250,000 HBV positive dads. These poor men suffer, nearly all have been denied protection for their children, I remember one week three of them called utterly desperate their children are a pin prick away from HBV. The inevitable infections are heartbreaking. We now offer the vaccination ourselves.

Hepatitis B Mom Vaccination Guidelines for baby factsheet

What if I test positive for Hepatitis B while I am pregnant?
Although most women do not have any pregnancy complications as a result of HBV infection she should be referred to a liver specialist for further evaluation.

How can I protect my newborn from Hepatitis B?
If a pregnant woman tests positive for Hepatitis B, her newborn child must be given the first dose of Hepatitis B vaccine on Day 1, Day 30 and Day 60 with a booster at one year. If a baby does not receive these injections, then there is a high possibility that he or she will become chronically infected. However if on the rare occasions the vaccine does not work do not panic rigorous blood precautions by the mother can still protect the baby.

How do I protect my child if another family member is infected with Hepatitis B?
Babies and children can be exposed to HBV from an infected dad, sibling, or other family member living in the same household. This can occur through contact with infected blood and bodily fluids. Vaccination is the best prevention against spreading the Hepatitis B virus.

Can I breastfeed my baby if I am infected with Hepatitis B?
According to the World Health Organization (WHO) it is safe for an infected woman to breastfeed her child. All women with Hepatitis B are encouraged to breastfeed their babies since the benefits of breastfeeding outweigh the potential risk of transmitting the virus through breast milk. In addition, since all newborns should receive the Hepatitis B vaccine at birth, the risk of transmission is reduced even further.

How can I prevent getting HBV if someone in my household is infected?
We recommend that anyone living in a household with an infected family member should be vaccinated. This is especially important for babies and children since they are at greatest risk for developing a chronic infection if exposed to HBV at an early age. Until your 3 injection vaccine series is complete, it is important to avoid sharing any sharp instruments such as razors, toothbrushes, or earrings, etc. since small amounts of blood can be exchanged through these items. Also, infected individuals should be careful to keep all cuts properly covered. Blood spills should be cleaned with gloves and a 10% bleach/water solution. Hepatitis B is not transmitted casually and it cannot be spread through sneezing, coughing, hugging, or eating food prepared by someone who is infected with Hepatitis B.

Remember that the best protection for you and your loved ones is the Hepatitis B vaccine. Over 1 billion doses of the vaccine have been given, making it the most widely used vaccine in the world!

Chapter 9 NHS & Overseas Healthcare Risks for HBV & HCV

Still even in 2015 our NHS dialysis, transplant, c section and surgery patients from before 1992 have not been safety tested and are not coming forward for testing; this is the challenge, and at once our greatest, gravest risk.

With the passing of Dame Anita Roddick, it becomes important to really focus on the NHS Hepatitis B and C Epidemic in terms of saving lives. To stand up and finally take note of the toll this virus can exact and think of the generations exposed to this most important danger. In particular, to see that with a 20-30 year lag during which the virus does its damage, we may have and should expect hundreds of thousands of long term undiagnosed to be at high risk. This will be a group most at danger towards retirement, their key risks will be the normal toxins alcohol, medicines (6% of A&E admissions are drug reactions) and obesity. Dame Anita Roddick was an extremely intelligent woman, yet even she was not able to achieve a test and diagnosis until needing a liver transplant. There are hundreds of thousands of caesarean section mums and post simple operation survivors who have run her risk.

Why do NHS Procedures from before 1992 need a HCV test?

The NHS admits 1 in 39 of its surgeries caused HCV before 1992.

Because Prison Blood was used massively until 1986 accounting for 70% of Hepatitis C NHS Infections, the HCV infections for surgery dropped from 2.6% to 1 %, with its removal. Because before 1992 NHS Hepatitis B and C infection was called transfusion hepatitis as it was very common, with 150,000 patients still infected and undiagnosed.

Basically, contaminated blood and blood products were components of dozens of standard medical procedures. Below data from the national blood sera bank (PHLS) reveals the Bulk of Infections are from before 1986 or from NHS Care during its period of using prison blood as a mainstay for supply.

Make no mistake every hospital in the UK, the USA and France used and infected patients with local prison blood up until 1986. So much prison blood was in use that it took four years to stop the practice in the UK. Many nations phased the practice out in the early 1970's after HBV was found in blood.

Because a test costs £1 and a liver transplant £100,000

Healthcare Infection Callers

Boy infected in London 2013 by kidney drain

Girl infected by NHS transplant 2007

Granny infected in Wales 2012 by gastroscopy tube died within 10 weeks fulminant. Hospital in cover up mode until previous patient with the gastroscopy tube was diagnosed HBV high load.

Police man Infected by NHS transfusion in 1980 after being stabbed denied travel costs to speak in the Commons, disgusting. Liver Cancer.

Patient Diagnosed same day GP felt reason was on file as transfusion HCV to distressed to speak knew nothing about HCV, sent info on HCV and Skipton Compo form stage 2, forgotten with non a and non b for 25 years like me. This is the norm, they have never checked the 30,000 on file as non a and non b.
Pilipino Infected via NHS and very ill from medicines poor Info on epilim chrono, talked about softer meds my relative has same problem improved

Lady HBV positive Ex husband and father dying in Canada shocked the Canadians said don't come unvaccinated while the GP said don't bother, arranged accelerated vacs explained blood hygiene told them to hug hold hands and kiss him goodbye Tears all round
Wife Watched her husband die, extended agony his eyes were black at the end, feel all stakeholders should see him, preventable if we had tested them Transfusion HBV on file.

Mum, son died of HBV just rang to see if anything would ever be done
Wife NHS infection needs compo poor guy is end stage HBV has none
Man HCV positive HIV positive from clotting factors Drug Reaction liver failure Feel this 2 liver failures on prescriptions in one day is the tip of a huge iceberg 1-200,000 people statistically suffer this. Given double dose blood thinners, aspirin and antiacid, GP did not check his other doctor's advice rushed to st marks and off the meds. Two liver failures due to GP prescriptions in one day

Factor 8 victim Just one visit to a liver spec in decades knows nothing about hbv Explained dangers of meds and alcohol and transmission Sent pack to Action Group and Lord Morris and patient
Kenyan Blood transfusion Stigmatised Sent info tears

NHS Surgery before 1992 was 1 in 39 HCV infectious

Surgery is the reason behind most (85%) of transfusions and also therefore most of healthcare HCV infections in the developed world, the US admitted to 200,000 HCV infections annually when using our Red Cross system of taking blood from prisoners 1945 -1985, we burnt the transfusion records instead. So unfortunately in the UK most pre 1992 surgery patients seldom consider or know whether their surgery involved a blood risk. In fact, nearly all major surgery involves 3-4 Units of blood and all surgery had a high risk of contamination before 1992. Testing is recommended for any minor surgery needing general anaesthesia and blood also. Basically, if you have had surgery in the UK before 1986 it is probable that you ran a 2.6% or 1 in 39 risk from the blood alone, with extra risks from clotting factors and immune globins depending on patient type. After 1986 the risk was 1% per transfusion until 1992. Hundreds of thousands of patients were infected before 1992, yet unlike France and the US our elders have never been safety tested.

The prevalence of HCV in England and Wales. kbalogun@phls.nhs.uk

OBJECTIVES: To estimate the background population prevalence of Hepatitis C in England and Wales, observe the prevalence over time and assess the extent of infection outside of known risk groups. METHODS: Sera from residual specimens from adult patients submitted to laboratories in England and Wales were tested for HCV. Testing was carried out using a pooling strategy.

RESULTS: The prevalence of HCV was in 1986 1.07%, in the multivariable analysis, prevalence did not vary significantly between the 3 periods 1986, 1991 and 1996 (P=0.14). The prevalence of infection was higher in males than in females (P=0.0013). An age-period-cohort analysis revealed a cohort effect due to a lower HCV prevalence in the most recent birth cohorts, that is, those born between the calendar years 1971-1975 and 1976-1980.

CONCLUSIONS: The majority of HCV infections in England and Wales were probably acquired before 1986. Infections in younger males identified in 1996 may signify more recent acquisition by injecting drug use.

Why NHS Transfusions before 1992 need Hepatitis tests

From 1945-1985 the NHS performed an increasing 200-400,000 transfusions each year. Below is the report that 2.6% of these surgical transfusions were Hepatitis C infected. These 5-13,000 Hepatitis C infections a year add up to a total of 250,000 surgery transfusion post-war infections. Or one in two hundred of us in 1990 as appear in the 1999 WHO Atlas. Globally 200 million people still have Healthcare Hepatitis C. With estimates of only 12 million active street injector HCV infections globally, you see the truth more clearly.

HCV is the largest Healthcare Super Bug Outbreak in human history first (250 million infections), and a street injector problem second (12 million infections).

Below, the devastating NHS infection level of 34% in mixed patients is admitted, yet it was decided to test only those patients who had run risks after 1988. The hundreds of thousands infected from 1945 to 1988 from prison blood have simply never been warned. Leaving several million at risk as Lord Morris puts it, "The Greatest Disaster in NHS History."

Below an NHS admission operations before 1992 was 20 times more infectious than a one night stand with HIV. (1 in 40 and 1 in 800 respectively) Alone on Earth our UK politicians decided it is not worth testing this NHS risk or mentioning it was often a worse risk in overseas healthcare like the US. This stupidity is a lot more dangerous than the HBV & HCV infections themselves.

Surveillance of HCV in England and Wales 1996
mramsay@phls.co.uk
In 1993 people tested between 1990 and 1993 revealed that the prevalence of HCV was highest among recipients of blood or blood products 34% and injecting drug users 67% and lower among other groups. In a study in early 1995, the prevalence of HCV was **2.6% in those transfused before 1985 1.0% in those transfused after.**

The pitiful UK effort above found only 2000 post 1988 infections and was the entire UK look back HBV HCV warning and testing campaign. It reached 2-4% of those infected.

Why NHS C-sections from before 1994 need a Hepatitis Test

Even with Anita Roddick's high profile celebrity death from c-section infection, the NHS has still not screened its pre 1992 C-section mums or publicised the role of immuno agent Gammagard. 400,000 thousand mothers have risked HCV from a C-section via the product Gammagard.

Baxter Healthcare Corporation, announced it was removing its immune globulin intravenous product Gammagard from the market worldwide because of the possibility that it may have transmitted the Hepatitis virus, including Hepatitis C. Baxter's IGIV is also named Polygram.

Anti d Globulin infects over a thousand mothers in Germany Gamma globulin contains antibodies obtained from blood donors. Although intramuscular use of immune globulin has not been associated with Hepatitis C in the United States, intravenous immune globulin transfusion has been implicated as a risk factor for Hepatitis C. In East Germany, 14 batches of anti-D immune globulin were contaminated with Hepatitis C. 1,018 East German women were injected from 1978-79 resulting in 76% Hepatitis C antibody positive in a twenty year follow up study10. The relative role of immune globulin in Hepatitis C transmission remains controversial. Since the mid-1990s, the U.S. military has shifted to a longer lasting Hepatitis A vaccination and the role of immune globulin has been limited. FDA 1994

Anti d Globulin infects over a thousand mothers in Ireland Ten years ago on this day, the Irish Blood Bank first admitted that some women may have been infected with the Hepatitis C virus from contaminated Anti-D, a product given to certain women in childbirth. After a huge political controversy and two Tribunals of Inquiry the true scale of the scandal emerged and shocked the country. Full confidence in the Blood Bank has yet to be restored. Over 1,000 women were found to be infected with the Hepatitis C virus. Around 90 people have died arising from the scandal. A voluntary reporting system remains in place, run by the Blood Bank itself. In a legal battle, the chief of the Blood Bank was suspended in 2002 and secured a settlement when the Blood Bank decided not to pursue the case in the High Court. A docu-drama No Tears was broadcast in 2002.

Alert to Blood Transfusion Service Board - 1991 The Blood Transfusion Services Board is alerted by an English hospital to the possibility that the six 1977 women cases may be linked to its "Anti-D" blood derived agent. Alert is disregarded.

Why NHS Blood Products before 1993 need a Hepatitis test

Canadian prevalencing of HCV would see these blood products comprising 15-20% on top of our transfusion infections. We use these products in identical ways and similar amounts e.g. Clotting and Immune Boost Products etc. There are dozens of conditions that were treated with these products 1945-1994 and during that time most carried an infectious HCV threat. Bearing in mind the sheer amount of blood products administered, see the Blood Products Laboratory brochure extract below, many, many more conditions were treated than just Haemophilia and C-Sections.

So if you think your treatment may have included a blood product before 1994, demand a HCV check. Few GP's are prepared to go through your file completely, so it is good to make a list of treatments including those from babyhood, and ask if there was a product or transfusion risk. The volume of these products used is clear from the Blood Products Laboratory below.

Every year the following products provide treatment

5,000 kilos of albumin are used each year in hospitals for the treatment of burns, shock and major trauma.

2,000 kilos of intravenous immunoglobulin is supplied to UK patients with immune disorders, including 1,800 patients with primary immune deficiency that requires an injection every two to three weeks throughout their lives, to protect them against infection.

120,000 bottles of anti-D immunoglobulin are used each year to protect unborn children suffering from haemolytic diseases of the newborn. This affects around

64,000 pregnancies a year and, in a small number of cases, can cause stillbirth, severe disability or death after birth from anaemia or jaundice.

25,000 vials of specific immunoglobulins offering protection against a range of diseases such as Hepatitis B, tetanus and varicella zoster. Alpha 1 Acid Glycoprotein, has been granted ods.

BPL has been using USA-sourced plasma since 1998 as part the Government's vCJD risk-reduction strategy. The USA has no cases of BSE"

Why pre 1992 NHS Dialysis needs HBV & HCV testing

Quite simply Dialysis may save lives but it desperately needs a HCV Safety Check when finished. 30,000 people a year need to know this fact. If you have had dialysis anywhere get your HBV & HCV Check immediately.

Dialysis Patients are now routinely HBV vaccinated.

Once again UK prevalencing and comprehensive testing of Dialysis HCV is poorly published. The last line of the report features the UK's failure to test these obvious high risk cases or even properly note their infection levels.

Report from the European Dialysis Treatment Association (2000).

Background- The high prevalence of Hepatitis C virus (HCV) in dialysis patients has been known since the early 1990s but its evolution over the last decade is poorly documented.

Methods- Chronic Dialysis patients from units from eight European countries, whose prevalence of HCV patients had been studied in 1991–1994 (and published except in one country UK of course), were tested in 1999.

Results - Prevalence also decreased in the participating units from

UK	7–3%	(at least 18,000UK HCV infections 1982-92)	
France	42–30%	Sweden	16–9%
Italy	28–16%	Hungary	26–15%
Belgian	3.5-6.8%	Germany	7 to 6%
Spain	5 to 12%	Poland	42 to 44%

Conclusions - The prevalence of HCV in Dialysis has decreased markedly over the last decade in the participating units from most European countries. A reduction in the prevalence of HCV patients on Dialysis has been mentioned [9] previously, on the basis of the 1992 and 1993 European Dialysis and Transplant Association registry data reporting prevalence's of 21 and 17.7%, respectively [1,21

Indeed, the prevalence was calculated in units 'testing most or all Dialysis patients for HCV'. In 1992, the proportion of such units was as low as 48% in Finland **or 29%** in UK.

Why NHS Transplants and Tissues need HBV & HCV Tests

To date there are reports of UK Transplant materials not being fully screened for HBV & HCV, at over 10,000 risks a year a lot of testing is required.

Before 1992 the problem with transplants was also compounded by the possibility of not just the organ being infected, but the blood to put it in, the blood products to keep it in and the large amount of injections involved often all being infectious also. In the UK between 1 April 2006 and 31 March 2007:

- 3,086 organ transplants were carried out (1,495 donors involved).
- 949 heart, lung, liver or combined heart/lungs, liver/kidney, liver/pancreas or heart/kidney transplants
- 2,137 patients received a kidney or pancreas
- 164 combined kidney/pancreas transplants took place.
- At any one time around 8,000 patients are waiting for a transplant.

Tissues

In the UK, human tissues and cells from both living and deceased donors are transplanted in an increasing range and number of operations.

- In 1993/94 it was estimated that some 10,000 procedures in the NHS involved a human tissue transplant. This is likely to be a considerable under-estimate of current usage.
- In 2005 3819 corneas were donated and 2622 grafts were grafted
- Other tissues and cells which may be transplanted include skin, heart valves, tendons, cartilage, gametes and stem cells, amongst others.
- Around 2,100 haematopoietic stem cell (bone marrow) transplants are carried out annually.

The study by Peffault de Latour and colleagues provides important insights into this problem by careful follow-up of 96 HCV infected survivors for up to 28 years. The cumulative incidence of cirrhosis was 24% at 20 years after transplantation, a remarkably high figure in comparison to the progression of HCV infection in non transplantation patients.

As many as **35% of survivors** from transplantation surgeries from before 1992 may be infected with HCV. All survivors, particularly those from transplantation surgeries before 1992, must be tested for anti-HCV and staged by biopsy for extent of liver disease if infected. This is easier said than done. Some people are lost to follow-up. The first step toward preventing the development of cirrhosis, however, is to emulate the practice of the Paris group by tracking all survivors and determining who is infected by HBV/HCV.

NHS Infection Numbers – with WHO model used globally

By 1998 Canada had found and tested most of its transfusion survivors, nearly 75,000 people. It has fully acknowledged an equal number may have died already from HCV complications over the past 5 decades of transfusing.

They admit a 0.4 per blood unit infection rate. They spent 3 years legally on the 3 models below to estimate hospital infections. Our Records state a 0.6% per blood unit HCV Infection Risk. We transfused 2 times the population.

Canadian Persons Surviving mid 1998
Summary of point estimates of HCV infected transfusion recipients

	Transfusion Infections		Blood Products Infections	
	Estimate	Limits	Estimate	Limits
Model 1	34,800	26-45,000	21,000	16-29,000
Model 2	36,000	25-49,000	24,000	19-31,000
Model 3	45,000	29-67,000	19,000	23-34,000

The Canadian Common Sense Healthcare HCV Prevalencing for Lawyers above would count over 100,000 in 2015 for NHS Survivors.

If Canada had 60,000 survivors we with double the population had 120,000 then add in we admit our blood was more infectious and we had 180,000 Survivors in 1998.

It's now about 100-120,000 with the above method and HBV added.

The UK has commissioned no comprehensive HCV prevalence studies on its dialysis, organ, c-section or surgical transfusion cohort's, either on their infections or deaths; such studies form another basis worldwide in estimating national infection levels. Here we are still using 90% error guesstimates and since 1996 have managed to avoid prevalencing HBV or HCV nationally. This cover up to avoid compensation is still going on legally. The nation is not vaccinating its children or testing its 15 million at risk, exactly because its health service is still in court claiming HBV and HCV infections never happened.

Prison Blood

I remember working in St Mary's Hospital in Paddington, upon my induction I remember noting the blood van went to Wormwood Scrubs for our supply. I would see them off every week making sure the entire hospital was full of blood mainly from heroin addicts, who always donated the bulk. Only St Marys and one other UK hospital ever tried to warn their patients subsequently.

The collection of blood from prisons and borstal institutions in the United Kingdom continued right up until March 1984, despite repeated warnings that the practice is unsafe. WHY did the Authorities persist with taking blood from prisoners for so long?

Here is a list of just some of the ignored warnings regarding UK prison blood:

In 1958, there was an early warning from a respected international source. Dr. J. Garrott Allen discovered what he referred to as the "prison effect" after conducting a survey in the Chicago area.

In 1980 we know that blood from Scottish prisoners was used in NHS transfusions despite serious concerns being raised.

Then in 1983, the Medicines Inspector commented adversely on the practice of collecting blood from prisons and borstal institutions.

By July 1983, the Medicines Division's Inspection Action Group had expressed serious concerns about the collection and use of blood from borstal institutions and prisons.

In the Nineties when the world realized that healthcare had globally infected 1 in 40 humans with HCV and 1 in 10 with HBV, we destroyed our transfusion records and forgot about "Transfusion Hepatitis" testing. Sadly some 3-400,000 HBV and HCV healthcare infected overseas victims have arrived since.

Most have joined our UK cohorts in ignorance and missed their safety tests and vaccinations since arrival to the UK.

Chapter 10 Drugs and HBV & HCV Risks

In the UK today great strides have been taken and real progress made at diagnosing, vaccinating and treating the nations injecting addicts and general prisoners for both HBV and HCV. HBV vaccine coverage in prisons is good and all addicts are also vaccinated and when necessary treated. Things are so good drug dependency wards are now less infected 0.7% than child wards 0.8% nationally. That said 5% of the worlds HCV, some 12 million infections have happened to those who Illegally Drug Inject and 1% of HBV, some 5 million HBV infections have also happened from sharing Drug Injecting syringes and equipment. As with healthcare HBV and HCV infections the group at greatest risk of death are the users from before 1992 who may now be 30 years away from their last risky illegal injection and not coming forward for safety testing, or simply quite unaware of the risk.

All Injection Abusers (even once) need a HBV & HCV Test.
In the wrong hands unhygienic syringes are a very deadly weapon. If you have ever injected anything outside a prescription from your doctors, even once, decades ago, even if you feel well, you need a Hepatitis B and C Safety Test. Injection Abuse clean needle centres report that many street injectors are using steroids these days, the risks are also quite real from blood stained crack pipes and snorting straws. As long as you have an injection habit, viral hepatitis will await you, so get into a programme to never inject or addict again. People living with addicts are at high risk from needlestick usually, and many get infected as they are usually refused vaccinations. Heroin can be notoriously fast acting, as passed out with syringe in hand or even arm images testify. HBV vaccination is the only protection for a needlestick risk.

Illegal Injector Calls (Intravenous and intra muscular self injecting is illegal because 1 in 10,000 can die from anaphylaxis without adrenaline)
Heroin Injector 15, HBV from sharing needles, bright positive and quick to assimilate HBV means great vaccs and meds and no liver problems. Children also need to know how a billion people caught hepatitis from injections,
Heroin Injector 17, sharing needles again until we teach blood hygiene in schools how can children realise the danger. Sharing razors, tattoo pins, compass games, chap sticks, bloody teeth, blood brothering, fighting all are blood risks every child must know. We warn them about matches and dog pooh, but blood, ooer!
Steroid Injector, 19, HBV outbreak, sharing at a gym. You can literally see the steroid injector abuse in most gyms now

Chapter 11 Genital Mutilation and HBV and HCV Risks
FGM practising nations have the highest level of HBV infection globally.

The FGM victims are testing across the world at 5 to 10% having lasting incurable HBV infections and 50 to 95% having had the infection at some point. It is extremely important people realise HBV is more likely to kill and 100 times more infectious than HIV. Victims are 1% dying by 20 and up to 20% dying by 50. One drop of HBV blood on a ritual razor can infect 10 girls a day for month. For under fives with childish immunity systems this equates to one cutter being quite able to incurably HBV infect 150 girls a month. Over the years we have spoken too hundreds of victims with healthcare consequences, we note that when survivors go yellow with Hepatitis afterwards, in Somalian it is termed Agbarshoe and in Kurdish Zereck. For tens of thousands of UK Nineties and Noughties survivors testing is urgently needed.

The 14 FGM Complications Factsheet

It is crucial to get FGM mums to relate their illnesses to FGM The highest maternal and infant mortality rates are in FGM-practicing regions.[17] One quarter of women in Central African Republic and 1/5 of women in Eritrea reported FGM-related complications.[20] Where medical facilities are ill-equipped, emergencies arising from the practice cannot be treated. Thus, a child who develops uncontrolled bleeding or infection after FGM may die within hours.[21]

Immediate Physical Problems

1. **Intense pain** and/or hemorrhage that can lead to shock during and after the procedure. A Sierra Leone study found that nearly 97 percent of the 269 women interviewed experienced intense pain during and after FGM, and more than 13 percent went into shock.[22]
2. **Hemorrhage** can also lead to anemia.
3. **Wound infection**, including tetanus. A survey in Sierra Leone showed that of 100 girls who had FGM, 1 died and 12 required hospitalization, 10 suffered from bleeding and 5 from tetanus.[24] Tetanus is fatal in 50% of cases.[25]
4. **Damage** to adjoining organs from the use of blunt instruments by unskilled operators. According to a 1993 nationwide study in the Sudan, this occurs approximately 0.3 percent of the time.[26]
5. **Urine retention** from swelling and/or blockage of the urethra.

Long-Term Reproductive and Health Complications

6. **FGM survivors are 5-10% HBV infected** – often the same unsterilized instrument is used on several girls at a time, increasing the spreading HBV or another communicable disease.[35]

7. **Problem menses**. In a study, 55.4% women in Somalia, reported abnormal menstruation.[27]

8. **Recurrent urinary tract infections**. A 1983 study in the Sudan revealed that 16.4 percent of women who had the operation experienced recurrent urinary tract infections.[28]

9. **Abscesses, dermoid cysts**, and keloid scars (hardening of scars).

10. **Increased risk of maternal and child morbidity**. FGM Women are twice as likely to die during childbirth and are more likely to have a stillborn child than other women.[29] Among 33 infibulated mothers all required extensive episiotomies during childbirth, second-stage labour was 5 times longer than normal, 5 of their babies died, and 21 suffered oxygen deprivation because of the long, obstructed labor.[31]

11. **Infertility.** In the Sudan, 20-25% of female infertility has been linked to FGM complications.[32]

12. **Some researchers describe the psychological effects** of FGM as ranging from anxiety to severe depression and psychosomatic illnesses.[33] Many children exhibit behavioural changes after FGM, but problems may not be evident until the child reaches adulthood.[34]

Complications Often Need Expensive and Ongoing Medical Attention

13. According to a study conducted in a small rural village in Sierra Leone, **83 percent** of women who had undergone FGM would require medical attention resulting from the procedure. [36] In Kenya, almost **half** encountered women with chronic FGM-related complications.

FGM often Impedes Women's Sexuality

14. FGM destroys much or all of the vulval nerve endings, delaying arousal or impairing orgasm.[38] In a 1993 Sudanese study, 5.5 percent of women interviewed experienced painful intercourse while 9.3 percent of them reported having difficult or impossible penetration.[39] Of 1,545 Sudanese women who had undergone the operation interviewed. Fifty percent of them said that they did not enjoy sex at all and only accepted it as a duty.[40]

Burkina Faso has led the way regarding both policy and successful elimination for the whole African Continent since 1990. Understanding their 25 year usage of each of anti FGM's 4 wheels is crucial as all 4 have created an incredible drop from **76% practising to just 9%** supporting FGM in 2015.

The 4 Wheels that end FGM in an afternoon

1. **Education** of health and birth consequences, Every FGM survivor needs the 14 points in hand and on all maternity and GP walls when deciding against it Every couple diagnosed with FGM present in the mum during maternity has a human right and huge need for to the 14 morbidities factsheet and knowledge of the laws and penalties to empower them.
2. **Laws**, our police to instruct parents at schools if it occurs they will be prosecuted, parents are responsible for making certain their child is safe.
3. **Penalties**, Each child cut £5k fine with age 5 safety checks for girls at risk. Obviously the penalty absolutely must hurt more than the cut. Cutters need 14 years no parole. They will have killed. Penalties are to fund the c-sections.
4. **Girl Human Rights** education for religious and community leaders who support the Practice, with jail for those thereafter caught advocating it.

Senegal and the UK are the poor examples in the FGM eradication league both nations need to do more with laws, health education and penalties. Senegal's poor drop from 26% practising and still 17% supporting, is almost as bad as us, wherein for decades almost no one has done anything for these poor agonized children.

Not one prosecution by July 2015 and tens of thousands of girls risking death and infertility and still we have wards full of maimed jaundiced girls actually getting younger every September. Forgive me but every FGM mum I have spoken to on the helpline was fast to learn and filled with care for their children. Given the facts and helped to teach others I trust them all to be out there eradicating the practice, especially former advocates of the practice.

Preferring politically correct silence to the eradication successes in other nations from 1990, for 25 years we have not enacted the systems to protect little girls from terrible pain and harm. Basically in 1990 we warned our surgeons to stop transmitting hepatitis with prison blood and pointless appendix and tonsil operations but we were tongue tied by politics when all these poor little girls and their mums needed news of simple medical facts and advancements. It is every girl's right to be safe from this in 2015.

Chapter 12 Sex and HBV & HCV

HBV & HCV Co Habiting Transmission
Firstly in relationships and Co Habiting situations it is important to remember non sexual transmission routes are the most common. Most co habiting household HBV (65%) and HCV infections (100%) are from shared razors, domestic violence and general blood spill accidents. The fact that 3 times as many siblings catch HBV as Partners reveals that non sexual transmission from a partner is the most common route. Many partners even after diagnosis are not advised of the main routes of transmission. Shared razors, lack of plasters, poor blood spill hygiene and lack of latex gloves are common calls and reasons for infections.

With HCV heterosexual transmission has never been documented
to have happened as it is only infectiously present in blood. The Results of a 10-Year Prospective Study by the US Journal of Gastroenterology found in 2004 no Evidence of Sexual Transmission of Hepatitis C among couples, With anal sex HCV transmission has been recorded among HIV positive gays.

With HBV when and how is it sexually Infectious?
Sex is a means of transmission with HBV as 15% of the infected will have high viral loads wherein the HBV is present in the sexual fluids. For instance approximately 4,000 migrant young mums are diagnosed with HBV each year during routine NHS maternity testing and we find only 15% of partners have the HBV infection or signs of having had it too. This is true of HBV positive mums who have had many children and been with a partner for decades.
The science behind this is that HBV can be infectious in sexual fluids as well as blood sometimes when the viral load goes above about 200,000IU/ml. This normally happens when acutely or just infected transmissions happen. Like many bugs including the common cold HBV is most infectious during the first 3 months. A recent caller was a St John first aider who caught HBV and by the time she went yellow she had a load of 30 million and had infected her partner sexually. So if a partner has HBV see if they know their individual risk level ask are they
- a low risk trace known to be sexually un infectious?
- un infectious, with undetectable results from Anti Virals?
- A high load needing condoms and your accelerated vaccination?
- Having an e antigen and getting more infectious?

These facts can guide and help a lot here, becoming NO or LOW RISK are important medical events in patients lives and affect partners a lot also.

Sexual Helpline Call Themes

One Night Stands Many calls are from people after one night stands who have read HBV & HCV can take from 2 to 6 months to show up. We have only had one who tested negative at 2 months test positive at 6 months since we started the helpline in 2004 is the point we make. In 5 years only one tested positive.

Oral Sex Many calls relate to oral sex, this seems common in Stag and Lap Dance venues, so the baffled virgin groom to be often calls, we even have call surges after TV shows and we have to say never recorded to have happened. Which is all we know about oral sex and HBV & HCV, neither the helpline or medical studies have noted infections via this route.

Anal sex however is definitely more of a risk due to wounding and bleeding possibilities. With transfusion Hepatitis B and C remember wound gateways are always hugely more risky than ear, vagina, and mouth etc gateways. Gay men are noted to be more infected with HBV due to this.

Saliva Sex saliva has not been documented to transmit HBV, however, blood from any wound will, so bleeding gums and lip cuts are times to not kiss.

University Sex One Phenomenon of Helpline calls is Fresher's, every year some 700,000 people go to our universities and seemingly have a huge amount of extra sex, tattoos and co habitation while often intoxicated. This population is more the world in one place than the UK in many campuses, so Hepatitis can be very present and we have still not tested enough to know what our students are dealing with.
So every October end we notice a rash of students who have caught HBV calling with symptoms or diagnosis, none have accessed any HBV or Blood Hygiene information at all. With 1 in 20 humans having HBV and it being sexually and co habitingly available, surely the students needing warnings and vaccination options should have some? Again students are often in serious debt and unable to access £300 vaccinations.

HIV Patients are immuno compromised and for this group HCV and HBV present a huge problem both viruses seem sexually infectious to this group. It is worrying how little they know about viral Hepatitis too

Hiding HBV can be a risk, and partners can retreat into fear and silence when finally told, especially when weeks or months have passed. Only honesty and vaccination seem to heal these, all patients should have the HBV Vaccination Schedule in the Vaccination Chapter to give Prospective partners.

Ultimately Viral Hepatitis is not HIV, with HBV a vaccine solves the sexual question, with HCV it is not a sex disease at all, you have to have two wounds, because it is a blood virus that's only transfusable. However HBV has the awful NHS choices "100 times more infectious than HIV" typo still on it and therefore many patients struggle to know how to warn prospective partners. We have noted cultural ways of doing this over the years of calls.

Inscrutable Silence
in the East. Chinese and Far East Asian ladies diagnosed in maternity over 13 cases have never revealed their HBV status until diagnosed in maternity. This culture of silence is common in the Far East, where for years before vaccination, HBV infection would be ostracized by communities,

I have a human right to tell no one Silence
in the West. There is a liberal they should wear their condoms attitude getting common, at my last help group 4 HBV patients had 4 years of unannounced sex between them, this hardly seems fair when there is a sure fire vaccine at the local chemist.

Blissful Optimism Silence
in Africa, Middle East and South Asia many may even remember going yellow but are unaware the virus is still in them, they may even like the Author have transfusion hepatitis on their file for 25 years like me and just not know.

All three silences overlook HBV has excellent medicines and vaccinations and they do lead to more sexual risk and infection.

Bangkok
Every year we get lots of Bangkok calls, thousands fly to somewhere where 80% of local people catch HBV especially to practice transmission routes, paid for sex, piercings, dentistry all unvaccinated. Even a brain dead fish bashed to a pulp in a liquidizer can see mandatory vaccinations for this destination are a good idea, but not our health ministers and health commissioners? One infection costs 20,000 vaccinations.

HBV & HCV Sexually Orientated Helpline Calls

Without info people with sexual risks just die inside as they google. The term 100 times more infectious than HIV and in saliva could have been written to send any nervous people raving mad quickly.

It is crucial to remember that HBV is 3 times less sexually infectious than HIV, a several thousand to one risk from a one night stand.

Assumption of transmission is the mother of all chaos

1. **Gay** 21 year old HBV positive had anal sex with 16 year old and HBV infection resulted. Father rang gathering hate mob ready to kill, gay man had been to GUM before sex for full set of tests but they forgot HBV, which is all too common. GUM clinic results confirmed things calmed dad as best no one understood only acute, he cleared.

2. **Young man** Stunned by HBV cleared diagnosis he had lived in Thailand unvooo for 0 months and was convinced HBV is a sex disease. He took a "which bitch" approach first he blamed his Thai girl for cheating and infecting him she tested clear then he accused his UK girlfriend even more convinced she was being unfaithful to him, she was clear also. He lost both girls but finally understood Thai tattoos a bad idea and the clear risk.

3. **Greek** Diagnosed 08 jaundice 03 Poor chap has wife whose vaccination don't work so he thought no wife and kids for 3 years and had a breakdown Doesn't understand rising load and low risk reassured will live long and vacc will work. Now getting engaged and Bosnian fiancée vaccinated.

4. **Nigerian Husband** tested HBV positive at work and was told, a low risk infection common with Africans mentioned to the wife at breakfast. After NHS choice reading she hit him with a frying pan when he got home.

5. **Husband** white British with Chinese wife positive, family in uproar GP not vaccinating parents. No one understood she is very low risk, no one explained she is fine health wise either

6. **Ghana** Diagnosed in Ghana and thought not true as often tested for things here had been to a GUM clinic many times, yet 15 years of unprotected everything sent info trained her up very receptive really got the hang of being positive Ghanaians so far are all like that

7. **Woman** Has had 4 separate GUM clinics STD check her. She has 20 years of unprotected sex with HBV on her conscience now GUM's have got to up their game on this and recommend every single gay for vaccination and African and pacific rim if we are to control the sexual spread

8. **GUM Nurse** Advised she is now low risk and non exposure prone asked can she stop condoms after 10 years as hubby vaccinated. I mean if a GUM nurse doesn't understand vaccs to the point of missing children?

9. **Chinese wife** diagnosed recently family not vaccinated again poor GP advice, sent info and vaccination schedule, I wonder if GP's fail to recommend the vaccination rather than say they do not actually offer the service?.

10. **Woman visits** partner yellow in ICU fulminant full of tubes, she is offered a leaflet saying 100 times more infectious than HIV, she had had sex with her partner the day before she rang in panic thinking he is dying and she will be full of tubes next and thinking the entire hospital had gone mad husband given no info but had a phone google to add to the chaos terrified himself Sent info explained results

11. **Asian man** 7 months failed to clear talked out of leaving family and into vaccinating them

12. **African lady** Thought she would die young and couldn't have a partner or kids, common Explained what a great 50 years I've had

13. **Ghanaian Lady** Had sex during menses didn't tell partner previously had not infected partner of 7 years, was told low risk by specialist no info on blood hygiene common problem explained honesty and vaccination

14. **Above's partner rang** Calmed him low risk tested clear sent info for both about liver health

15. **Man** Sexual risk sent nuts by internet explained HBV is less sexually transmitted than HIV sent Info arranged vacc booking

16. **Mum in law** Denied vaccination live in son in law has HBV greater families even siblings are almost always ignored, told her to tell walk-in clinic and say she's a swinger. She was vaccinated. She is a real character

17. **Man** Dating new girl who knows nothing about her HBV, no GP sent info. There are 2 million from endemic areas without GP's.

18. **30 year old lady Imam** Diagnosed at birth mum was positive too. Lost her notes told not infected now has hubby and 3 kids to test

19. **mum and daughter** have signs of developing liver disease planned test and vacc for hubby kids and lesbian lover, explained her low load state sent info about attendant ailments

20. **Man** HBV Positive condom broke arranged test, utter terror.

21. **Lady** Pakistani finance tested positive GP told his girl HBV is probably sex or Heroin problems told her 45% of Pakistanis catch HBV and to test his extended family for the other infections found a mum and sister, sent info arranged vac saved arranged marriage.

22. **Carer** Diagnosed in June 5 months later has no idea if she going to die, has lost partner feels could never have a partner Sent info built hope told work not to keep vaccination shots going

23. **Man doing anal sex** while HBV positive no info or referral never told GP advised blood hygiene & condoms & referral sent info

24. **Greek scared** Had blow job advised no risk and value of status awareness see appendix.

25. **Mother in law** Infected son in law confessed to adultery, he was Nigerian so probably from childhood as other lady tested negative. advised partner child vaccinations sent info

26. **Man OCD** Ran sexual risk in Thai un reassurable many calls. NHS HBV information actually creates OCD patients.

27. **Man** Really suffered poor info "the 100 times more infectious a kiss kills granny type" GP variables in explanation again. Reckons we saved his life sent info

28. **Man** Diagnosed HBV & HCV via phone no advice health visitor then told neighbours his HCV was mis diagnosis GP assumed IDU no referral wife left due to no vac and he tried suicide Support and Info

29. **Gay man** Ran risk never heard of HBV or the vaccine advised vaccination and tests

30. **Man** Ran oral sex risk had test and spent 3 years thinking he had HBV told him his results meant clear sent to GUM clinic where he finally realised he was clear

31. **Man** Terrance Higgins Trust referral partner infected with bad liver tests alts needed more info drawing the Trust Higgins Trust close, they have about 20 million more than us annually

32. **Gay man** Ran sexual risk told get tested and vac sent info. Far too many gay men are unaware they are supposed to be HBV vaccinated if they are active sexually.

33. **Man** Poor liver tests, sex risk with prostitute, got tested, infected

34. **Polish Friend** Her friend got chbv in 1999 came to the UK thinking it's over GP just mentioned she is high risk a lot of migrants think it goes away with onset symptoms and ignore the problem, just like me. Told her go back to GP and demand referral liver function tests and scan Husband refuses test as he thinks he's infected now. For 5 years her GP has seen her diagnosis and not advised her.

35. **Woman** Her Partner developed HBV 4 months ago during her unprotected sexual relationship with him. Bleeding anal sex involved. People planning rough anal sex need vaccinating. She should be lucky this time she is getting final test in December sent info

36. **Wife** CHBV husband keen to learn sent info In touch

37. **Nigerian** 6 years of UK sex no protection GP mentioned condoms not vacs for sex, this is just too common why not vaccination and ask if married. Arranged vacc for wife.

38. **GP** HBV positive wife GUM clinic told him after 3 shots failed to do 1 in a year. Often GP's simple lack of English is the problem, from GUM to dumb, arranged 3 shots privately as risk is high, condoms fall off. I mean our GP's are calling a helpline to vacc their own selves now!

39. **Man**18 HBV blood tests 3 Cognitive Behavioural courses 6 months of terror. Had run no HBV risk solved in 5 minutes chat. The NHS spent the equal of a year's funding for our helpline on him.

40. **Lady** HBV+ needed all the usual kit Engaged and positive about things Just love empowering patients and the I am going to be fine at the end, so few patients understand their infections.

41. **Lady** Positive but poor vacc info thought kissing was infectious for many years. Sent accelerated schedule Just an accelerated schedule so helps imagine asking a date to wait 9 months for a kiss

42. **Gay man** Recent infection, so many are not vaccinated Sent acute advice and fingers crossed

43. **Mum** Son dating a Romanian HBV positive girl he has trouble getting vacc Arranged they felt all they could do was condoms It is best to get partners to study up HBV together and use that info to increase love then vacs get easier n understood by the by

44. **Man** Just diagnosed sent pack and vacc schedule he was not told to vacc girlfriend unless we give vacc schedules how do they know what to do?

45. **Nurse** Wife asked Is HBV hubby faithful by GP and told forget kids calmed wife and him, his uncle and cousin infected so common among Turks

46. **Bulgarian lady** Emotionally isolated and depressed no understanding every visit to unit destroys her we trained her up with HBV positive she is just stunningly pretty started dating

47. **Bulgarian** Just diagnosed so upset about a sexual infection Mother also has it so explained how it gets from brother to sister and mother to child and in Bulgaria mainly from healthcare. Explained care path and HBV positive she felt much better so many people have such preconceptions HBV is HIV

48. **Gay man** Is vacc safe for in this order blow job anal sex and giving blow job anal sex said yes his score will make him safe, a voice said I told you so, laughter frolicking noises man said "I really have to go."

49. **Asian man** Went to lap dance club and a ladies naked down there touched his willy for a second during a dance   Definitely no risk! Explained he is not at risk from this brief down there touch recommended vaccination lap dance clubs bewilder many patrons

50. **Man** Woke up next to African girl after office party married shocked did not remember if he did or how he got there recommended super low risk and vaccination

51. **Wife** Husband HBV from Africa wife told a sex disease by GP pointed out Gambia endemic wife tears of relief other family siblings infected HBV positive training referral not offered arranged

52. **Lady** Infected Turkish hubby told HBV is like having flu London GP did not understand chronic and acute HBV googled for an answer in front of patient said he had only had 1 case in 13 years means he has never tested anyone and his local maternity is 1 in a hundred

53. **Turkish** girlfriend awful alts 500 and symptoms poor info using condoms not vacc Checked meds alcohol and diet found was McDonalds manager changed food symptoms gone normal alts

54. **Indian** Infection from back home knows infected but out of meds Tenofovir and out of care 3 years. Panic tried to get into care taught what HBV is to him, explained HBV positive and got GP and referral tears. Too many migrants have no GP or healthcare access

55. **Spanish lady** Just diagnosed googled for an hour had bottle of wine and rang explained low risk sent pack explained to partner should be fine he was clear

56. **Pakistani** HBV positive poor understanding depressed and no future wife attitude explained HBV vac and dating. 2 weeks later he is getting married it's amazing Pakistani parents have wives up their sleeves for their sons at the drop of a hat

57. **Lithuanian man** infected mother of 6 high load and fulminant, ICU case in semi coma from blood toxins. Then a BBV Nurse shook her hand and with a clip board asked if she was paid for sex

58. **Gambian Nurse** Left in limbo for 5 months was clear in 2009 and diagnosed in 2011! Knew nothing about HBV or transmission Hospital still vaccinating her!

59. **Woman** wandered if handshakes infect Sent info

60. **Woman** asked if swimming is infectious after a HBV person swims in the pool, explained water borne and cholera to her

61. **Fresher's Teenager** Wanked and anal fingered man 2 days previously recommended struck by lightning risk in the absence of any wound arranged vaccination she understood status awareness

62. **Man** One night with a Chinese girl called 9.04 Sunday morning status chat get vaccs at GP

63. **Uni Outbreak** Boy 19 pretty depressed, with globally 1 in 30 sexually active humans having HBV, we need to tell our students the risks.

64. **Mother** Son infected at uni suicidal isolated, he thought a kiss could kill and didn't know of vaccination schedule, sent info.

65. **Mother** Son infected in uni fresher's left with bad info and pretty depressed, kids know nothing about this vaccine nothing, sent info explained how we have wives, children, travel and health etc, tried to make him feel he has a future, explained he is like me infected at 19 30 years ago. **Above's mum** rang and said he's going back to university and is a different person made donation

Chapter 13 Getting Hepatitis B & C Tested

The Hepatitis Pre-Test Discussion

Gets informed consent for testing from the patient after explaining

1. Printed HCV/ HBV information about the annual global deaths due to poor diagnosis. The value of knowing liver status.
2. Assessment of Infection Risks and or Symptoms that need testing, Explanation of risks for HBV/HCV being 1 in 3 humans common.
3. Information about confidentiality and the notification process. Very rarely insurers and employers may access this information, so arranging insurances or work issues if you are e.g. a surgeon or a boxer can be important.

On Occasion it is necessary, to assess support for a result, e.g. children, mentally ill and the elderly, and to reduce infection risks, e.g. vaccination/safer injecting/sex/blood hygiene.

The Hepatitis Post-Test Discussion

Should give the test result in a manner that is confidential, sensitive and appropriate to mental state, personally, covering

1. An Understanding of HCV / HBV's Disease Journey. With HCV explain it is not a sex disease but a Super Bug Pandemic affecting 200 million
2. A Liver Friendly lifestyle, explain how HCV/HBV kills with pills or alcohol
3. The Basics of both HBV Vaccination and Blood hygiene precautions, people need to use plasters and bleach spills. HBV also requires safe sex as that virus is in sexual fluids
4. Medical Referral to a liver specialist and a source of disease information, such as the Hep C Trust or Hep B Foundation, for the person's discretion.
5. Assessment of mental state, I've seen people diagnosed with liver cancer and months to live and be very sensible and people diagnosed with a normal life expectancy and no damage have a breakdown and need a psychiatrist.

On Occasion it is necessary to arrange Rehabilitation or Psychological counseling or therapy.

Hepatitis B test results Factsheet

A simple blood test can detect if you are infected with the Hepatitis B virus. If infected, tests check on the viral load of infection, measured from 0 to 2,000 as uninfectious, 2,000 to 250,000 as low risk 250,000 to 1 million as medium risk, 1 million to 1 billion as high risk. More tests help us see if the infection is active, or a new acute clearable one. Further liver tests can assess if and how active the virus is and if it may cause harm or infection. As all the HBV positive Premiership footballers and Olympic athletes' have reported HBV positive individuals normally have nothing wrong with them, it is the above tests that play a key part in confirming this.

Hepatitis B Blood Test Results

HBsAg	positive	**Lasting Infection**
anti-HBc	positive	
anti-HBc IgM	negative	
anti-HBs	negative	
HBsAg	positive	**Acute Infection**
anti-HBc	positive	
anti-HBc IgM	positive	
anti-HBs	negative	
HBsAg	negative	**Susceptible**
anti-HBc	negative	
anti-HBs	negative	
HBsAg	negative	**Immune due to cleared infection**
anti-HBc	positive	
anti-HBs	positive	
HBsAg	negative	**Immune due to vaccination**
anti-HBc	negative	
anti-HBs	positive	

Tragically very large numbers of NHS GP's and staff struggle to interpret these most complex of blood results. We have constant calls from them requesting help with this. Many patients are being left with the notion they actually have Hepatitis B when they do not or told nonsense that a cleared infection can reactivate by GP's. Above the readings of "Immune due to cleared infection" is often seen as an infection. E.g. Mid Staffs took 4 weeks to tell a Consultant with this result he was not infectious. He needed valium to cope with the worst moments of his life, callers have been left misdiagnosed for decades in many cases, many have forgone partners and children and lived shadow lives without any real access to facts.

Acute Hepatitis B Factsheet

The main reason HBV is child hepatitis, is that a baby who catches HBV will 95% of the time not clear it, an under 5 will 50% not clear it and a child under 18 will 25% not clear it. Adults need to remember 95% of the time they will clear HBV, we note those missing sleep, on alcohol and antibiotics are the ones that struggle to clear.

With an estimated 14,000 plus catching HBV each year we get many calls from the just infected and diagnosed. These poor souls are often battered by symptoms especially jaundice, brain fog and utter exhaustion as they try to understand hepatitis. It is crucial they understand that 95% will clear the HBV virus, many get depressed hit the bottle or take pain killers and give themselves a lifetime infection. The acute infection is a about 6-7 month cycle from infection to clearance and if ever there was a time when zero alcohol, zero prescriptions and zero fried foods and a 2 litre water jug and lots of sleep was needed I promise it is these 6 months. Below the HBsAg and HBeAg is the HBV and the anti HBc and anti HBe are us fighting with anti bodies.

Hepatitis B Timeline

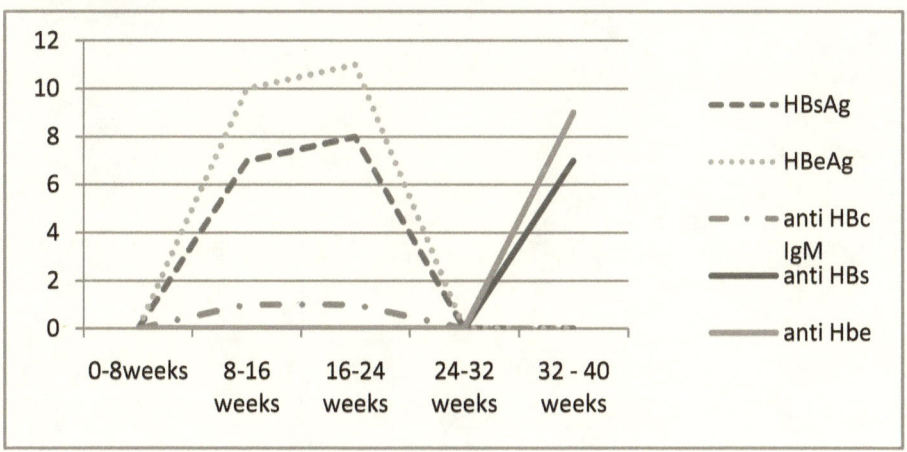

Above after 6 months the e antigen or HBeAg (the increasing part of HBV) is killed and hopefully the s antigen or HBsAg (the virus itself) is killed also. 95% of adults then produce the anti HBe and anti HBs antibodies and clear at six months. The anti HBc IgM is present until the virus clears or becomes permanent. If you are one of the unlucky ones to not clear, always remember the diagnosed early on are never left to develop liver disease these days and with vaccination all will be well.

Chapter 14 Getting Hepatitis B Vaccinated

Hepatitis B Vaccination factsheet

- The standard course of immunisation is 3 injections over 6 months on Day 1, Day 30, Day 180.
- Adults who need protection quickly can have a schedule over 28 days. Day 1, 7, 28. The vaccine is administered intramuscularly, usually into the deltoid muscle[3], a booster at 1 year is recommended. It can be used in those who are immunocompromised, as with HIV infection, but a higher dose may be required or extra booster injections, with HIV beware of CD count drop.
- Babies have 5ml half doses at Day 1, Day 30 and Day 60 with booster on 12 months.
- An accelerated course over 2 months is possible for combined Hepatitis A and B vaccines.

The vaccine should be given into the deltoid region or anterior thigh in babies. It is less effective if given into the buttock. It is quite possible that a course may give lifelong immunity,[4] but for health professionals one further booster at 5 years* is recommended. Antibody titres must be tested in health professionals 1 to 4 months after the primary course.

- A titre above 100 mIU/ml is regarded as adequate.
- Around 10-15% of adults fail to respond to three doses of vaccine or respond poorly.[1]
- Poor responders with titres of 10 to 100 mIU/ml should have a booster and those with a titre below 10 mIU/ml should repeat the course.
- Those over 40 years old, who are obese or who smoke are more likely to fail to respond.
- Alcoholics are also reported as having lower seroconversion rates, particularly those with advanced liver disease.
- Patients who are immunosuppressed or on renal dialysis may also respond less well and require larger or more doses of vaccine.
- Failure to produce any antibody after 2 complete courses should not be seen as necessarily meaning no immunity, as immunity to the disease is largely cell-mediated rather than by antibody.

*Of a thousand people vaccinated and having no boosters 3 became infected after 10-15 years. 5 years is chosen due to safety, health care workers are not suddenly "at risk" after 5 years. Many returning to work after 15 years get infected though.

Chapter 15 Should we vaccinate all children for HBV
And just how at risk are they?

A key reason for writing this book is to get into the public domain just what we have been experiencing on the National HBV Helpline regarding calls from children infected and ongoing risks that they are facing. Every parent and child has a right to know the virus is infectious in their schools and the simple facts about how it transmits and is becoming a growing risk, especially in our multi cultural cities.

Prevalence of child HBV in our Hospitals NHS figures

Child Wards	(10,121 tests)	General Wards (110,464 tests)
2008	0.5%	2.5%
2009	0.9%	1.8%
2010	0.8%	1.6%
2011	0.8%	1.6%
2008-2011	0.7%	1.9%

The above testing reveals our children are testing 35 times more infected than their US counterparts. With hospital figures at 0.7%, actual street and school prevalence will be 0.35% as most developed nations see a halving of numbers from ward to school due to wards having more likelihood of having ill children on board and children with hepatitis present more often. Still at 0.35% it is by far the worst outbreak in the developed world. A one in 300 incurably afflicted rate. It is easy to see why globally every single nation with endemic HBV communities vaccinates all their children at birth.

The figures above instead of being proclaimed and leading to universal vaccination of all newborns and catch up vaccinations for older children in every UK school as in 200 other nations, have been archived already by the by politicians at the Department of Health. We feel the NHS and BBC have no right to hide these facts and healthcare from the generation who need them.

It has been decided that people should simply not know ever how much HBV is infecting our children. Which leaves millions of children and parents completely at risk and unwarned, imagine our adults, 1 in 650 get HIV and we have a 30 year uproar, our children test for HBV at a 1 in 300 rate for 4 years of testing in 22 hospital centres across the UK and almost no one even knows and HBV is a better killer of people these days too.

Onward HBV transmission rates among children

Having seen the scale of infections, the next step for parents is to study where and how and how often our children are catching HBV. How onward it is among those at risk, so being a migration nation we can look at the US to suggest an article to explain how onward infectious HBV was among US children before it rolled universal HBV vaccinations. Their example is ideal as the US is closest to us in demographics. The article below explains how the US has avoided 500,000 under 16's catching HBV since 1990.

> **US 2001** - Childhood HBV Infections before Immunisation
> Results. Annual rates of infection ranged from 1 child in 40 (2580 per 100 000) in children of Southeast Asian origin to 24 per 100 000 in non-Asian children. Before vaccination HBV was annually infecting 16 000 children who were younger than 10 years.
> Conclusion. Thousands of US children were infected each year with HBV, before routine infant Hepatitis B immunization, placing them at high risk of death from cirrhosis or liver cancer.

A 1 child in 40 annual rate was noticed among US Chinese migrant children. A scale of sorts is visible the more infected the parental generation the higher or lower onward transmissions among children. So we find migrant children in the US had these rates and it is public knowledge there, we also find so many migrant NHS staff callers who have experience of HBV are just horrified at the lack of protection. Large numbers have experience of childhood HBV infection already in the family. So what have we seen in the UK when testing children in the UK in communities, starting with an African 5.7% HBV infected parental population.

> **UK 2002** - HBV prevalence Somali households in Liverpool
> Results A study in the Liverpool Somali population to determine the prevalence of Hepatitis B markers. A total of 439 subjects were screened. It was found that 5.7% of had HBV. Seven of 80 (8.7%) children born in the UK and aged 5 years or less had evidence of having had HBV. Only one mother had HBV, this suggests horizontal transmission continues at an early age among Somali immigrants. Conclusion The UK is one of the few western European countries which has chosen not to comply with the WHO recommendations for universal Hepatitis B vaccination.

A 1 child in 50 annual rate is actually about normal for a 5.7% population without access to care, warnings or vaccinations and it has become politically normal to just pretend otherwise. The real problem with having no proper prevalencing in our schools is that 30% of UK children now live in endemic communities and go to local schools; we see 90% of calls from highly mixed schools.

To guide parents here it is worth noting that when in 1999 it was admitted that UK prisoners where 8.7% having HBV markers it became mandatory to HBV vaccinate them all. Yet when we saw the same rates in migrant under 5's we have done nothing for 12 years. Even now at the Trust we are allowed to train prisons in HBV testing and vaccinations, yet school nurses dealing with outbreaks we are still not allowed to help by governors and principals.

The understanding seems wholly missing that these children are catching HBV and that is of course what happens until vaccination in their communities. We are avoiding a maternity mum to new born infection but have simply not comprehended that HBV dads are twice as infectious and outnumber mums by 2 to 1, that HBV siblings are 3 times more infectious, that journeys home are infectious. We are avoiding the basic facts that HBV is 100 times more infectious to children than HIV and these children and the epidemic are concentrated into local schools. The next article focuses on a 2% HBV infected parental UK community from the Indian Sub Continent.

> **UK 2003** - Hepatitis B among UK South Asian children Results. 9% of total HBV infections were in children under 15 years. The most frequent source of infection for South Asian children under 2 years of age was within the household, 45% of infections in South Asian children less than 2 years were reported to have been acquired overseas.
>
> Conclusion. Our study shows that Asians are at higher risk of HBV while resident in the UK, particularly in childhood, suggesting that **significant transmission** during childhood may occur among UK ethnic minorities from high or intermediate prevalence countries.

Nine per cent of the 500,000 people with HBV in the UK add up to 45,000 UK children catching HBV incurably since the millennium. Armed with this grim information in 2014 our charity asked 14 questions of the Health Minister via the office of Sir David Amess Head All Party Commons Group on Hepatitis about these 0.7% HBV infected children on our wards, the 40 schools and dozens of infected children and the thousands of adults infected as children we have heard from.

She replied she cannot recognise the published figure of 0.7% of children being HBV infected or imagine that migrants are 3% HBV positive either. Our calls for a child prevalence study and promptly rolling universal vaccination unfortunately sent her off nagging our patients below, discovering half our HBV kids (20,000) are UK born and tragically 1% dying by 15.

> **Feb 2014** prevalence of diagnosed childhood HBV mramsay
> Analysis estimated 448 diagnosed HBV cases (prevalence, 4.6/100,000) 328 cases revealed that
> - 1% had ESLD, (2 cirrhosis and 1 liver cancer)
> - 50% UK born, Pakistani & Chinese making up half
> - 50% born overseas, mainly Africa and E Europe
>
> concludes that horizontal transmission among UK-born children was identified in only 3 children born since 2001, the prevalence of diagnosed childhood HBV is low, although the number of undiagnosed cases is difficult to estimate.

She ends with a mindless 3 HBV horizontal (means adult to child or child to child) infections and no idea of if we will ever know more. I mean 28 families and children bravely volunteered their experiences to warn others and she mentions 3 to them. They worked so hard to create a slide presentation email for the minister and 25 of them are told they still don't exist.

The point for parents is we are experiencing an entirely predictable and preventable boom in HBV infections in our children. They have a human right to know the World Health Organisation urges them to get vaccinated. These children need help, underestimating HBV and blatantly refusing to safety test our schools for 25 years, has left thousands infected, at risk of serious illness and, as is tragically clear above, 1% dying at 16.

Our Most Incredulous calls are from Doctors denied Child Vaccines

Specialist in Blood Sciences I asked my GP to HBV vaccinate my girl of two and he denied the risk. I have personally studied onward HBV spread among thousands of children in rural China several years ago. It is just incredible to me that a man in his profession should not know the need for this vaccination. I am new to this country and dread to think that all Chinese suffer in silence without this vaccine for their children.

Rumanian Doctor, she asked her GP to vaccinate her baby was told not at risk. Just plain incensed, could not believe a GP is unaware kids catch HBV. She had seen yellow children in her pediatric ward in Rumania for years. She had vaccinated 3 other children in EU.

Polish Nurse denied vaccination just couldn't believe it really panicked herself her sister has HBV, she believed no one could forget HBV these days and as is common thought the word hepatitis in the Red Book was HBV not just a Hep A shot. She lost faith in her GP she had her child vaccinated in Warsaw.

Care Home Manageress has 3 HBV patients' elderly frail who have young visitor's usually grand children. After seeing an 11 year old with blood on his hands after a dressing fell off she advised the family to get vaccinated. GP denied risk and the 5 vaccinations.

Manager at a large HBV Vaccine Manufacturer met at conference for HBV, mentioned he has vaccinated his big daughter back home in new Zealand and realised he had not vaccinated the little one. From Dover to Auckland the children are all immunised at birth except here Mr Manager had not been able to access a vaccine for her here. Here where she schools with the only unvaccinated endemic Afro Asian eastern EU children left on Earth. Their office ran 2 London marathons to raise awareness and funds for our work.

Dr Hashi from London, could not believe Somali children were tested in Liverpool and found 8.7% catching HBV and they did not prevalence more or vaccinate straight away, visited the office in shock to study the calls.

Dr Dadabhoy lecturer in Hepatitis at the Royal College of GP's we discussed the thousands of unvaccinated for HBV boys sent for cut throat rituals shaves in 3.5% HBV infected Saudi Arabia.

Dr Mann we discussed the enormous need for junior boxers and rugby players to be HBV vaccinated. For premiership blood hygiene to be taught.

Charlotte Leslie MP and Health Select Committee Member made time to understand boxing club infection reports and transmission risk levels and shared our concerns UK amateur boxers lag far behind others in obtaining HBV vaccinations.

HBV Trust - Having a minister who ignores WHO guidelines needs to become illegal, the 40,000 children consistently indicated to have HBV by our last 10,000 sentinel tests are definitely not going to be saved by people guessing their number might be 3. It is an insult to our 28 HBV kids question. We in the Appendix word our reply to this nonsense. Prevalencing is testing a few schools and learning how infected they are, not nagging the diagnosed.

Dr Phillip Lee MP bravely asked for border safety testing of endemic area survivor migrants and their children and was called racist for his concern. It is surreal how quickly people assume you wish to exclude the infected rather than diagnose and care for them. The Immigration Act will allow some 200,000 more undiagnosed viral hepatitis infected citizens to arrive without any access to the care they need over the next 10 years therefore.

Chapter 16 Getting Hepatitis B & C Care

Lifestyle counseling factsheet

GP & Support Group Do's and Try not To's

Do encourage liver good life, diet, attitude, vaccination, abstinence, education

Do print HBV Booklet with every diagnosis and explain results deeply.

Do vaccinate all partners and relatives (work sport colleagues often)

Do support the unhealthy livers with Treatment and any constant side effects

Do make clear HBV is only caught by those forgetting their vaccine

Do assume 80% of presenting infections are unavoidable and innocent

Do not prescribe long term unless effects are monitored for liver effect

Do mention 21 units creates cirrhosis do not say moderation like a killer robot

Do mention fried food and obesity doubles the danger

Do explain the healthy livers may not need treatment highlight they are healthy

Do not assume Injecting Drug User or sex risks try to find the risk

Do understand the billions at work childhood and healthcare risk

Do not call HCV sexual only transfusable

Do try, not mother to child, but Maternity Unit infections

Do teach & encourage Premiership Blood Hygiene

Do try to use simple terms for Hepatitis B results

HBeAg	Got it increasing	(high risk yet quickly manageable)
HBVDNA high	Got it increasing	(high risk yet quickly manageable)
HBsAg	Got it	(low risk and often left untreated)
Anti-HBc Igm	Fighting it	(6 month recent infection)
Anti HBs/HBe	Cleared it	(had HBV and are immune)
100 Anti HBs	Immunised for it	(had vaccination and are immune)

Just Diagnosed?

3 Aspects comprise a HBV/HCV care program

Lifestyle

Nothing affects our livers as much as our lifestyles. They basically have to cope with everything we throw at them. The big 3 to avoid are alcohol, obesity and medicines. The big 3 to make sure of are regular eating habits, sensible hydration and a healthy mindset. Don't be alone try to meet on message boards and helplines or groups before forming harsh ideas about hepatitis.

Monitoring

Make sure you get scans and liver tests lft's done every 6 months and that your GP is aware not to prescribe medicine that's hard on your liver. Remember HBV/HCV usually takes 20 years to damage a liver and then usually the unlucky ones who are obese, busy taking medicines or social drinking. If your infection is inactive like 80% are, modern medicare will give you a normal life span. This is extremely important to know and up to half of patient callers do not.

Intervention

For certain patients it is advisable to take anti viral medicines now available. These drugs are used to stop active infections harming us and they are now very effective. Having had hundreds of Just Diagnosed on the help line here is the advice patients and mums who've experienced being diagnosed and adjusting usually needed most.

General Emotional Advice

- HBV & HCV have effective medicines diagnosed before liver disease patients will be just fine these days
- Don't feel guilty, remember 1 in 3 humans have caught these bugs
- Don't feel infectious use vaccination and blood hygiene
- Many patients find HBV makes them live longer, healthier lives
- Try to learn about Hepatitis B or C, and how they are managed.
- Understand your level of infection, if it is low risk it is good to know
- If your liver is fine, you have a life of health to plan for, don't forget.

116

Watch who you tell?

- Do not announce HBV & HCV; people may react with ignorance.
- Let knowledge of your infection make a few relationships stronger
- Take time to understand things first and tell people who will learn also
- You will need to teach people what HBV or HCV is, very few know. This is the one where vaccination is far the most important precaution.

What to do next? Be Careful with toxins, ignorance and alcohol

Fried foods or oily and "ghee" type foods are all not good and can easily inflame the liver. If you already have liver inflammation, both obesity and alcohol increases the risk and speed of developing cirrhosis. Clinical studies have repeatedly shown that long term HBV/HCV infection and even moderate drinking can quickly result in Cirrhosis.

Real caution needs to be exercised with many medications also, it is important your doctors consider your liver status when prescribing each and every time. It is important to note that most HBV infections do not lead to cirrhosis or liver cancer, even after decades, this is clearly lifestyle related. For some it is only acute reactions to alcohol or medication or maternity testing that ever gets them diagnosed.

Unfortunately in the UK, GP's and NHS Choices are very poorly equipped for Hepatitis discussions. Most have poor risk understanding of childhood HBV or healthcare HCV, no HBV or HCV atlases of the 2200 million infected, no non stigmatised test risk posters, hepatitis booklets or factsheets have ever been given them.

They also call a lot with vaccination and test result questions and these are core areas of dealing with us hepatitis patients.

Sadly many NHS staff and therefore the public still look on mainly child HBV & mainly healthcare HCV as infections from drugs or sex as per the NHS information they have. By far the hardest part of being just diagnosed is actually ever understanding clearly what is viral hepatitis and if and how it is affecting my liver, far too many patients never understand for years basic facts.

Liver Function Blood Tests factsheet

Healthy ranges for Blood tests for Liver Function

ALT	0 - 45	U/L	
GGT	0 - 45	U/L	
AST	0 - 45	U/L	
ALP	30 - 120	U/L	
BILIRUBIN	0 - 20	U/L	or 0.174 to 1.04 mg/dL
ALBUMIN	38 – 55	g/L	or 3.8 to 5.5g/dL
AFP	20 – 32	g/L	or 2 to 3.2g/dL

ALT (alanine aminotransferase), is elevated means inflammation of the liver.
GGT (gamma glutamyl transpeptidase) is elevated means alcohol or toxins.
AST (aspartate aminotransferase) is elevated liver damage.
ALP (alkaline phosphatase) is elevated in liver and non liver disease.
BILIRUBIN is elevated, yellow eyes, tired, sweats, itching, brain fog
ALBUMIN falling levels of blood albumin show deteriorating liver function.
AFP (Globulin protein). Elevated in liver cancers.

These tests give an excellent insight into if our HBV or HCV is harming us yet. These tests 60% of the time show a liver that is managing its HBV or HCV problem well with no signs of harm. However in some patients regardless of actual viral load of HBV or HCV they will show the extent of liver hardship. It is very important to understand ALTs, many patients have a score of 46 and assume a dire fate awaits! The scale goes up to 2500 and a pint will be 50 for instance! These scores go up and down with every meal. With ALTs 40% of us have them a little up for years, from 65 to 125 was my score for 25 years, without being tested. These scores are usually controlled very quickly with anti virals these days. We also get calls from the HBV moms who have AFP's up a little, 5 or 10, before and after birth, and are terrified of liver cancer. A score in the hundreds indicates liver cancer whereas a tiny fluctuation is actually common for pregnant mums. We have noted Hepatitis patients have Alt scores with paracetamol over years of a 1000, we have had fast food cause 500, with alcoholics we recommend testing on Mondays after binges so they can see a several hundred ALT and often GGT scores showing damage. We often see perfectly healthy people with perfectly healthy liver scores who just have not realised they are in the inactive grow old and die of something else group! I remember one caller who spent all his savings expecting to die at any moment and we had to point out he had a barely there trace of HBV never known to harm or infect anyone. It is important to understand our liver function tests, inactive is inactive, often the patient never understands this good news.

Liver Scans and Liver Biopsies Factsheet

An ultrasound scan shows fibrosis, cirrhosis levels, cysts, gallstones, fatty accumulations and cancers. With imaging tests of the liver and gallbladder, we can determine the degree of liver disease if any, and whether the HBV or HCV did any damage initially. Liver scans often throw up terms that some patients can find new confusing and quite scary.

Liver Fibrosis
When Hepatitis B or C are in the systems for decades they tend to cause a level of fibrosis scarring. This is usually measured from 1 to 6 on a scale. The important thing for patients to remember is the liver has a lot of spare area to process our food and build us daily. Basically a liver can be 5 out of 6 parts damaged fibrosis scar tissue and work absolutely fine just like mine these last 10 years. What matters is whether the liver is performing its duties well, keeping us healthy and this is normally the case even with extensive fibrosis.

So patients need to stay calm as often callers have just been hit with the diagnosis of hepatitis, then to hear about serious liver damage can be very worrying when actually things are very healthy and life expectancy still quite normal. About 40% of patients tend to have some fibrosis usually at a 2 to 3 stage and once diagnosed medications and lifestyle changes can improve the liver and remove some of the fibrosis. I myself went from 5 out of 6 to 3 out of 6 over the last 10 years. Remember half a liver can be cut away and grow back within 6 months. Fibrosis is actually just a scar, made out of scar tissue and if you think about it scars do not harm people do they?

Liver Bridging and Portal Fibrosis
Most fibrosis forms along two axis on the liver around the portal vein thus portal fibrosis and across the liver thus bridging fibrosis. Neither observation on our medical files means an illness or even a loss of liver function. In cases of alcoholism the constriction caused by fibrosis can be problematic but other than that we have no helpline reports of any problems that fibrosis even advanced can cause.

Liver Biopsy
These are mainly done these days as a baseline for treatment with anti virals with both HBV and HCV. The biopsy allows the Liver team to get our problem onto a microscope slide and gives detailed information on the livers cells and can show up rapidly any subsequent changes to the liver while on medication.

The Palette of HBV Treatments - Factsheet

The goals and aims of HBV treatment are to lower infectivity and stop liver damage. This is because no drug is effective at removing the virus. Hepatitis B HBsAG on your test result means you are infected but you are a low infection risk and HBeAG means you are infected and the virus is replicating and you are a high infection risk.

Chronically infected individuals with persistently elevated ALT's, a marker of liver damage, and high e antigen or just HBV viral loads are candidates for therapy. Several medicines treat Hepatitis B. If you do not need to start treatment immediately, you will be monitored over time to know when hepatitis becomes more active. Once you start treatment, you will have regular blood tests to see how well the treatment is working and to detect side effects or drug resistance. Monitoring will continue after finishing treatment to detect signs that the infection has come back.

Each patient may have a different set of needs or treatments according to tho faotoro and thoir individual health, further these medicines evolve and improve rapidly, being on a trial is quite normal in this field of medicine.

1. Lamivudine — Lamivudine (Epivir-HBV®) is effective in decreasing Hepatitis B virus activity and ongoing liver inflammation. It is safe in patients with liver failure and long-term treatment can decrease the risk of liver failure and liver cancer. (See "Lamivudine monotherapy for chronic Hepatitis B virus infection".)
Lamivudine is taken by mouth, usually at a dosage of 100 mg/day. The major problem with lamivudine is that a resistant form of hepatitis B virus (referred to as a YMDD mutant) frequently develops in people who take lamivudine long term. Other medicines are available that are less likely to cause resistance.

2. Adefovir — Adefovir (Hepsera®) is an alternative initial choice for people who have detectable Hepatitis B virus activity and ongoing liver inflammation. An advantage of adefovir compared to lamivudine is that resistance to adefovir is less likely to develop. In addition, adefovir can suppress lamivudine-resistant HBV. (See "Adefovir dipivoxil in the treatment of chronic Hepatitis B virus infection".)

Adefovir is taken by mouth, at a dosage of 10 mg/day, for at least one year. Most patients will need long-term treatment to maintain control of the Hepatitis B virus. Adefovir is a weak antiviral medicine, and resistance does occur over time. Other medicines are available that are more potent.

3. Entecavir — Entecavir (Baraclude®) is generally more potent than lamivudine and adefovir. Resistance to Entecavir is uncommon in people who have never been treated with antivirals, but occurs in up to 50 percent of people who have used lamivudine. (See "Entecavir in the treatment of chronic Hepatitis B virus infection".)
Entecavir is taken by mouth, at a dosage of 0.5 mg daily for patients who have no prior treatment and 1.0 mg daily for patients who have resistance to lamivudine. Most patients will need long-term treatment to maintain control of the Hepatitis B virus.

4. Tenofovir — Tenofovir (Viread®) is more potent than adefovir. Resistance to Tenofovir is rare. Tenofovir is taken by mouth, at a dosage of 245 mg daily. Tenofovir is effective in suppressing Hepatitis B virus that is resistant to lamivudine, telbivudine, or Entecavir. Tenofovir is not as effective in patients with adefovir-resistant Hepatitis B. Resistance to Tenofovir is uncommon.

5. Telbivudine — Telbivudine (Tyzeka®) is more potent than lamivudine and adefovir. Resistance to telbivudine is common, and Hepatitis B virus that is resistant to lamivudine is also resistant to telbivudine. Telbivudine is taken by mouth at a dosage of 600 mg daily. Other medicines are available that are less likely to cause resistance

6. Interferon-alpha — Interferon-alpha is an appropriate treatment for people with chronic Hepatitis B infection who have detectable virus activity, ongoing liver inflammation, and no cirrhosis. Both conventional interferon and pegylated interferon are approved Interferon is given for a finite duration. Pegylated interferon, a long acting interferon taken once a week, is given for one year. This is in contrast to the other hepatitis treatments, which are given by mouth for many years until a desired response is achieved. Drug resistance to interferon has not been reported. The disadvantages of interferon-alpha are that it must be taken by injection and it can cause many side effects.

Finally, Interferon apart, the only side effect on the helpline is vitamin d deficiency, which leaves thousands of patients sad and tired. We advise multi vitamins with the anti virals and vit D testing every time for this reason.

The Palette of HCV Treatments - Factsheet

The Treatments currently available are successful at curing the infection in around 85% of cases. Treatment for chronic Hepatitis C usually involves using a combination of two medicines with Boceprevir for genotype 1 cases

Pegylated interferon (given as an injection) – a synthetic version of a naturally occurring protein in the body that stimulates the immune system to attack virus cells

Ribavirin (given as a capsule or tablet) – an antiviral drug that stops Hepatitis C from spreading inside the body

Boceprevir and telaprevir
Protease inhibitors block the effects of enzymes that viral cells need to reproduce good for genotype 1 The medications are designed to be used in combination with pegylated interferon and ribavirin

Course and dosage
The length of your recommended course will depend on which genotype of the Hepatitis C virus you have. If you have genotype 1, a 48-week course is recommended. For all other genotypes, a course of 24 weeks will be recommended.
Weekly injections of pegylated interferon.
Ribavirin is normally taken twice a day with food.
Boceprevir and telaprevir are tablets taken three times a day for 48 weeks.

How effective is treatment?
The effectiveness of combination therapy depends on the genotype of the Hepatitis C virus. Genotype 1 is more challenging to treat. 50% of people treated with combination therapy will be cured. Other genotypes respond better to treatment, with a cure rate of around 75–80%.

You have a blood test at 4 weeks into your course, and again at 12 weeks. If the test shows that the medications are having little effect in removing the virus, it may be recommended that treatment is stopped as further treatment may be of little use.

Newer more effective less toxic medications are about to come on stream so many patients are waiting.

HCV Side effects can be serious and are vastly worse than HBV

Side effects of combination therapy are common and can be severe as the ribavirin burns the blood away to get the HCV. Three out of four people being treated will experience one or more side effect.

Side effects of combination therapy include:

A drop in the number of red blood cells (anemia), which can make you feel tired and out of breath, loss of appetite, depression, anxiety, irritability problems sleeping (insomnia),difficulties concentrating and remembering things hair loss, itchiness, feeling sick, dizziness, flu-like symptoms, such as a high temperature, that occur in the 48 hours after an interferon injection

These mild side effects may improve with time as your body gets used to the medications. Tell your care team if any side effect is becoming particularly troublesome as your dosage may need to be adjusted.

The key hardship with this is your weaknesses get exposed, if you have previous conditions they go crazy, I remember a epileptic convulsing with every ribavirin pill, a cirrhotic getting a 50 million higher hepatitis load and 90% eczema, a patient needing 4 units of blood per 30 ribavirin pills. These can be unexpected and sudden serious deterioration side effects.

Further if patients are down 1,2,3 or even 4 units of their normal blood and would benefit from a transfusion they should at least be told.

Coping with side effects may be challenging, but it is recommended that you continue to take medication as instructed. Missing doses to try to minimise side effects will reduce the chances of you being cured. With far better medicines available soon I finally dare to mention I did half the treatment for half the 12 months in 2007 and cleared. I had seizures for 4 months and am photo phobic and limp ever since, but I am alive.

Health Risks after HBV or HCV Diagnosis

Hepatitis, Alcohol and Binge Drinking
Alcohol is approximately two to four times more destructive to the liver of about 1 million citizens with viral hepatitis. 60% of those drinking 21 units go cirrhotic after 5 years. Alcohol abuse is often fatal to the undiagnosed. One helpline caller had quintupled his ALT score with a weekend binge.

Hepatitis, Prescriptions and Binge Medicating
The following list is a guide to medicines used to treat many medical conditions. The list does not include all medicines that may affect the liver systems. If a medicine you are taking is not listed here, check with your doctor. One helpline caller noted an ALT score of 625 after 3 months of paracetamol. We had 3 callers in A and E one Christmas due to prescriptions, 6% of A and E admissions are due to drug reactions and we are convinced hepatitis patients are suffering terribly here. We have regularly audited patients parked on varied prescriptions that are literally making them very ill. A Norwich patient on painkillers had been to A and E more than 10 times and was still prescribed, an anti biotics for clamidiya caused another HBV patient to liver fail completely and they kept giving it to him until an ICU unit worked out it was killing him. Another patient was given paracetamol, he reported nose and bottom bleeds from week one and was prescribed for 4 years. **Audit with your liver team and GP anything you are on permanently, get both their numbers and use them, is advice we give to patients.**

Acetaminophen Paracetamol	Antacids
Antibiotics	Anticholinergics
Anticonvulsants	Antihypertensives
Antituberculins	Calcium channel blockers
Chlorpromazine	Colchicine
Iron	Laxatives
Nitrates	Nonsteroidal-anti-inflammatory
Potassium chloride	Protein Shakes
Quinidine	Theophylline

Hepatitis, Obesity, Diet and Binge Eating.
While not as yet totally defined, many factors influence the rate of disease progression. Diet likely plays an important role in this process, as all foods and beverages that we ingest must pass through the liver to be metabolized. In particular obesity and fatty liver disease can further damage the liver. Keep slim avoid fried food and late night eating as the liver heals when we sleep.

Transmission General Precautions Factsheet

If I am infected, how can I prevent passing on the virus to others?

This question happens down the phone with enormous intensity from the Just Diagnosed so we felt it deserved a page of its own. It is truly terrifying for people to be told they have HBV by a GP or Sex Clinic and check NHS choices all alone. There they read that HBV is 100 times more infectious than HIV and in the saliva, then they read creates liver cancer which is 99% fatal. Then of course they ring the helpline in their hundreds in a terrible state, it often takes months for them to get over it all and many never do.

A key suffering is the fear of having infected or infecting a loved one. Firstly we find it very important for the patient to realize that they are not an infectious plague but just their blood in contact with a wound is. Then we supply the gloves and scrubs blood hygiene training and the list of useful tips listed below. Most of all HBV patients need to realize many HBV moms raise babies who fail to vaccinate safely. To date I have not heard of such an infection over 11 years on the helpline, the precautions work. All mums are proper special.

These are general rules that thousands of families and patients found useful guides if you have a current Hepatitis B infection:

- Make sure partners and children are vaccinated
- Make sure all your siblings and parents are tested and vaccinated
- Make sure living companions, contact sports are vaccinated too.
- Use & Teach blood hygiene. If any of your blood spills, clean with bleach or hot water. Cover your cuts and offer plasters immediately.
- Wear latex gloves whenever dealing with others wounds
- Never share razors etc, and bleach clean items (work tools) that may be contaminated with blood.
- Use condoms until they have been fully immunised and have been checked to see that the immunisation has worked by a blood test.
- Avoid tattoos and piercing

To date 5 callers are tied on diagnosing 5 relatives, a Chinese, Somalian, Ghanian, Nigerian and a Pakistani. HBV is a family bug, I have not found an extended family with just one infection. Usually from a family of 5, four will have been infected and one or two will be chronic.

Diet to keep the liver healthy

Liver Health management is very much everything we eat and everything we drink, it is extraordinary how many hepatitis patients thought they were supposed to have right side pain when they have eaten and not been told to eat what does not hurt! I remember one Nigerian family, mum and teenager doing late night pizzas and fried chicken for years with all sorts of symptoms that went away. Tiredness bloated, nausea, foggy, right quadrant pain like a companion are all often poor diet. Drink wise we need 2 litres a day of water. It is amazing just how often people forget this, it is the method of the human body for working well. Just a 2 litre jug every day from the fridge as a ritual is very helpful for the kidneys to aid carrying away toxins.

I find nearly all callers especially our glorious HBV moms are quick to fully understand we all have to admit we have a liver situation and we can get smart in the kitchen or we will suffer the consequences. If ever there is a time to get out of a rut with food just after diagnosis is a great time. The callers with just infected children are the best at this, yet we all deserve this care. Go mashed potato, not chips, go oats not fried bacon and eggs, drink water, buy the foods that help you, give the wine rack away, throw out the packs of chemist pills. Remember HBV and HCV are often harmless by themselves; it is in conjunction with toxins that they become far more dangerous. 20,000 curries later is too late for many. About 70% of patients are very healthy with inactive infections that liver units do not prescribe anti virals to, it is however important these patients realise the diet is the prescription for all of them and getting it right is guaranteeing a longer than average life expectancy.

10 excellent foods that are liver friendly, aiding healing and building health are **Carrots, Beets, Green Tea, Olive Oil, Tumeric, Lemon Juice, Leafy Greens, Avocado, Milk Thistle and Spinach.** 10 sources of Plant-Based Protein are **Kale tempeh hemp seeds quinoa chickpeas broccoli tofu almonds lentils chia seeds.** While animal products may be high in fats, plant-based proteins contain a ton of good-for-you benefits like fiber and antioxidants that the animal foods lack. Plant-based foods like legumes, nuts, quinoa, hemp seeds, and soy are all sources of protein (and the last three are all considered "complete proteins" because they contain all 9 essential amino acids). We have callers who have high ALTs on protein shakes. Too much protein can lead to inflammation and is hard on your kidneys. How much do you need? Aim for 0.36 grams per pound of body weight. So if you're a 140-pound female, that's roughly 50 grams.

Diet for the Liver Damaged

Fat and Liver Damage
Fatty fried foods are very hard for the liver to digest, they frequently cause pain to longer term patients, creating fatty liver so should be taken rarely. Picture oil on water undigestable or grease in a drain, fat is already a killer and hepatitis makes it harder for the liver to process this highly processed toxin

Iron and Liver Damage
The liver plays an important role in the metabolism of iron since it is the primary organ in the body that stores this metal. The average diet contains about 10- 20 mg of iron. Only about 10% of this iron is eliminated from the body. Patients with Hepatitis B & C cirrhosis sometimes have difficulty excreting iron from the body. This can overload of iron in the liver, blood, and other organs. Excess iron can be very damaging to the liver. Patients with Hepatitis B & C whose serum iron level is elevated, or who have cirrhosis, should avoid taking iron supplements and restrict the iron rich foods in their diet, such as red meats, liver, and cereals fortified with iron.

Protein and Liver Damage
Adequate protein intake is important to build and maintain muscle mass and to assist in healing and repair. Protein intake should be between about 45 – 120 grams a day in patients with hepatitis, unless Encephalopathy occurs. Encephalopathy is an altered mental status. It has been shown that restriction of the diet of animal protein and maintaining a total vegetarian diet, helps reverse this condition and improve mental capacity. Advanced scarring of the liver or cirrhosis can lead to fluid in the abdomen referred to as ascites.

Salt and Liver Damage
Patients with hepatitis who have ascites must be on salt restricted diets. Every gram of sodium consumed results in the accumulation of 200 ml of fluid. The lower the salt, the better this fluid accumulation is controlled. Sodium intake should be restricted to 1000mg each day, and preferably to 500 mg per day. For example, one teaspoon of table salt - 2,325 mg of sodium! Most fast food restaurants are a no no. Meats, especially red meats, are high in sodium a vegetarian diet may often become necessary. Patients with hepatitis without ascites are advised not to overindulge in salt intake, although their restrictions need not be as severe.
We advise all callers with HBV and HCV to restrict vitamin pill use to one multi vitamin tablet a day, as iron and vitamin e can get to toxic levels.

Chapter 17 HBV & HCV and the Emotional Effects

NHS Information here is 25 years out of date there is not a family leaflet on HBV or HCV for the diagnosed, no one has ever mentioned HBV affects the same amount of humans and is just as carcinogenic as say smoking in decades! Our point here is 80% of callers are suffering from depression due to poor, little and quite unrepresentative facts. Yet nearly all our care is focused on their livers not their hepatitis education, 35% of diagnosed patients could not explain the difference between HIV and HBV, during one survey. Half said they had no idea of their life expectancy in another fully 80% agreed HBV is far more a mental social problem than a health one. Even our 50,000 HBV Mum families have not had one booklet or leaflet or poster produced for them. We have spent billions on smoking yet a half dead patient has to pay £100,000 to set up a charity and helpline to offer the UK any of the common warning materials for Viral Hepatitis, or a voice for patient, child and migrant infections. With HBV the inequality of service is just incredible, patients have wept just on seeing someone with a public tent with information and factsheets and booklets about it.

These poor people are diagnosed with something no one, including many NHS staff knows important facts about and they are very isolated, most never meet another soul with experience of HBV. We find most are quite alone for 4 months until they meet a liver team and by then the misunderstandings have happened and no further education happens. Information's written for heroin addict, gay, prostitute and prisoner charities are often causing more harm than good and NHS pages are just a mix up of them. The forcing of safe "How to have multiple sexual partners and practices" and "How to inject heroin safely" information and the hiding of the actual transmission routes usually leads to a life of shame and isolation to some degree. I mean the common cold is more likely to infect Junkies and Prostitutes but we know how we get it too. The fact is the President of America is proud to campaign for HBV, his mother's country is 85% catch and 10% keep the virus, and he will tell you so, yet here we have Boy George and Russell Brand who are proud to be quoted on hepatitis, neither are any use to our annual 8000 HBV and HCV mums diagnosed at 3 months pregnant or the 81"% of patients on our books who are just like Mr Obama's mum. I remember a caller fresh from NHS choices saying "Yeah he had the HBV you know, the gay one" This is where the Stigma comes from it is entrenched in NHS information, they have banned the HBV and HCV atlases, how can they or anyone know about hepatitis? Many patients think most of the others are prostitutes and criminals after reading NHS choices.

HBV & HCV and the Emotional Effects Calls

A Rumanian lady rang 57 from the excellent St Mary's Liver Unit with her results, unfortunately the unit decided to not print them for her. As she mentioned what she remembered yes her liver was functioning good, yes her scan was good, yes her response to medication is good and after 6 months she was out the door in a flash having seen yet another stranger doctor.

Point being it took one hour and twenty minutes on the helpline before I heard her laughing and feeling confident. No one asks us if we have found our HBV has ended our ability to find love, no one asks if we have confused ourselves with "I best not have kids." No one asks are we under the impression we may die in agony quite soon.

It is amazing a Unit I admire and am proud to have as a charity advisor, I know they have stamped successful undetectable for HBV ideal liver results excellent medicine compliance on her file and yet not asked her if she feels crushed by HBV! Anyway we found she had vitamin D zero levels tested recently at the GP and well this is the side effect of Tenofovir and creates exhaustion and sadness in people. Like many patients she has never met another patient. My experience of her level of deficiency of was utter exhaustion and sorrow; it goes the moment you get the vitamins.

Lovely Nigerian Mum rang 28 and just diagnosed with HBV. She was informed by her GP she is a chronic active super carrier of the virus with the S and E versions and should see a liver doctor quickly, he also informed her that she has kidney stones and gall stones and liver fibrosis damage. Mum opened a bottle of wine and started googling, times we hear this, anyway she tapped in chronic super carrier and something and came up with the USS enterprise weapon of mass destruction, chronic in the oxford dictionary added never ending and incurable. She looked at her son as someone already exposed to a lethal dose of deadly radiation and quarantined herself in the house. Then she read a normal infection is 100 times more infectious and worse than HIV, and being a super carrier she would imagine super means 100 times 100 then she read in the saliva and one drop of HBV can infect 100,000 units in a laboratory. At this point she gave up on how infectious she was and went to see a friend face mask on, more wine ready and they started googling and decided to study fibrosis and stones and cures.

First up was the letter box incision, literally as per the name sizewise, for the gall stones. Then the images for sound blasted blood stained kidney stone removals with kidney out options. The real blow was the fibrosis leading to liver cirrhosis and cancer and 1% chance of survival page. This sort of left a deep impact, 1%. Anyway pointed out level 3 fibrosis is fine and liver bloods fine, Tenofovir will have you undetectable for Xmas, gall stones need milk thistle, kidneys need 2 liters' water and lemon a day. Vaccinated son in time for University and job done. Why I am so confident with this one is I had kidney & gall stones same liver readings and way worse fibrosis 11 years ago.

Friend Could find no information with which to cheer a patient only 100 times worse than HIV and one toothbrush and you die sent info recommended vacc
Woman Had an infected friend couldn't find a single positive online comment so rang us, pointed out her friend should be fine Sent info
Husband Has cHBV Chinese wife and needs IVF poor fallopian problem, they have both been delayed for 18 months and now pct is ordaining a budget. The fact GP's forget how good we are at preventing baby infections every time they are asked is irritating there's a whiff of why should junkies have money to have poor in danger diseased kids. Rang IVF guru mailed IVF data
Man Diagnosed 3 days ago for accountancy post in Abu Dhabi then destroyed himself reading NHS websites very intelligent Masters in everything. Denied job utterly distraught thought had to be alone for life and world would see him as an addict, no info felt no one will ever hire him thank goodness he rang

Pakistani Acute. GP said after a google search just like flu nothing to worry about had gone quite nuts for 3 weeks and lost all faith in NHS Another GP looked up NHS choices decided with his symptoms liver cancer might be setting in. Patient was actually acute and needed our clearance programme
Mum Worried about son's depression and isolation after HBV diagnosis he is on Tenofovir explained HBV to him and uninfectious as undetectable Transformed himself went back to uni girlfriend.
Turkish mum Planning suicide rope around neck hysterical, baby wont vacc after 6 shots fell out of liver unit contact. Read 90% unvacc babies catch from mum so decided to kill herself before she infect baby. Calmed and calmed explained precautions to make sure baby safe tears of relief undid rope on tree in garden months of calls fine
Albanian Infected wife and cleared hubby GP made a hash of tests he sent patient to liver unit worried him half to death for a cleared infection wife left due to arguments about infidelity.

Ethiopian Diagnosed 4 years ago missed appointment fell out care shame was suicidal about low risk infection at first, common. No understanding HBV or transmission only got in touch due to NHS porter job. Lucky Ethiopia vacced his wife she is due over soon trained HBV positive and premiership blood hygiene did job app and refer letters sent info laughter and tears

Japanese lady Got top new York job at oil co in panic about declaring HBV she read out the obvious NHS says it is from drugs and immorality and 100 times infectious and in saliva How can an innocent child infection that can be easily managed get turned into such a monster in a half page of disinfo?

Really felt for her Pacific Rim just do not want to mention this stuff. Told her be a CEO, don't be hbv victim, tell them like 1 in 4 humans are infected and explain HBV is an easy manage bug and every global employer should know exactly how to overcome it in a workforce wherever on earth efficiently and cost effectively with excellent vaccinations and meds to become undetectable, add that the US president or chief executive is proud his family is also at the forefront of eradicating it in a generation. Imagine she can deploy rigs the size of cities that change per person wealth in nations and even she was struggling to find words to explain her infection. She got the job.

Indian said being diagnosed with HBV is like being told a story you just cannot follow I am a healthy carrier of a fatal virus, was where he gave up trying to follow. He has HBV and no help for years explained GP and liver unit's explanations of HBV as they went blah blah blah. He did not understand anything that was said to him spent 1 hour to teach what HBV is and why he will be fine via the 17 page booklet. This is why the just diagnosed pack is crucial a lot of people just don't learn well when meeting many individuals rapidly all doing new and strange things HBV & HCV bloods, lft bloods scans and biopsies, using words that nobody understands often.

Wife Husband returned from 5 months work and serious dentistry in Hong Kong HBV positive 3 weeks after return wife threw him out to garage. She mentioned hubby hung himself after 20 year's marriage I fear for her too. Pretty sure she understood GP meeting and assumption of sexual transmission was wrong. I have waited just 17 months on this helpline to prove what I thought after day 1 namely that the dis information out there is causing suicides. Her last partner cheated a lot. She changed GP.

Lady, 42, a musician was in a coma from acute HBV infection with alts at 2500, drifting in and out of consciousness full of tubes, fighting for her life with a viral load over a thousand million. Up pops a lady saying she is a BBV Nurse, with hard to grasp strong accent and form at the ready, after prodding the lady alert she asked her name address date of birth and If she is accepts money for sex, on replying no the BBV asked if she had ever been paid for sex, she said no looking at a interested male visitor opposite Then she was asked if she has anal sex, she said no, then the question had she ever had anal sex, cringingly she said yes and a large circle was drawn on the form. Section 2 smiled BBV leading with, do you sleep with other men as well as your husband, she said no and then, did you ever sleep with other men. She said yes and sorry and cried a lot and her machines began to wobble and the ICU removed BBV, an affair from 20 years ago when hubby left and came back had happened. Anyway next morning 9 am patient awakes and BBV is looking down. How was she and does she inject heroin, no, then did she ever inject heroin no. Smilingly Section 3 had she ever been unhygenically pierced or tattooed she crying again with 105 fever said she does know if she is filthy. Had she had unhygienic non sterile operations or injections overseas? Don't know. It was at this point that she cracked up and asked to be discharged from the ICU pulling out tubes and her husband rang the helpline.

This is the worst case of what is actually standard practice! BBV means blood borne viral diseases nurse and they are trained to vaccinate injectors, prisoners and prostitutes and fill in risk questionnaires in particular. We spent a week re writing the risks for HBV and HCV with a BBV nurse in Oxford once, he had run out of injectors to vaccinate and was completely unaware his town hosts a lot of the last unvaccinated for HBV universities on Earth. BBV staffs are quite unaware 2 billion innocent child and healthcare infections have happened. With HCV he had been told it was 95% from injecting when globally, ahem like Oxford is, it is 95% from healthcare and 5% from injecting.

The point here is patients seriously benefit from education and there simply is none for mums, children or staff with HBV. We are confronted with a Monolith of NHS aspects all trained and convinced many of us do not exist! All 800,000 of us with child HBV and Healthcare HCV. As Sir David Amess head Commons Hepatitis Task Force put it you mean children catch HBV? As Minister Ellison put it we do not see any migrant increasing UK HBV levels. Every single caller had suffered because of this BBV training at some stage, two callers termed them bloody bitch nurses due to their assumptions of heroin or infidelity and ignorance of the common child and healthcare risks.

Chapter 18 The Cost - Mortality and Morbidity are Booming

I think every Epidemic that infects billions and kills 100 million like viral hepatitis deserves a proper warning on the packet. Below is a list of the awful ways HBV and HCV can kill. There is no better reason to get tested. Sadly the NHS seriously under counts these deaths, with the US noting 20,000 France noting 4,000, we count just 370. Many staff are quite unaware just how deadly it is, thinking HIV is more harmful. The last HIV consultant I lectured with said he was saddened watching Hepatitis kill the patients he had saved from Aids anyway.

The Most Common Causes of Death from Viral Hepatitis
Reported to the National Helpline 2010 to 2015

Liver Cancer	Bile duct Cancer
Kidney Cancer	Cirrhosis Liver Failure
Non Hodgkin's Lymphoma	Wildenstein's Disease
Skin Cancer	Strokes
Prescriptions Liver Failure	Suicide

We contacted Cancer research UK to ask is anyone counting the tidal wave of HBV HCV deaths from Hepatitis Bile Duct, Kidney, NHL, Skin and Blood cancers and stroke, liver reaction drug failure and cirrhosis deaths. They said no and mentioned they are lowering their guesstimate of HBV and HCV liver cancer by 70% making them 3 times less deadly here than anywhere on Earth!

It is easy to see how from 8,000 annual deaths with hepatitis and about 2500 because of hepatitis, we have just 370 on certificates.

This is where the Spin kills, as we pretend away 25 years of infections and deaths, GP's are still saying "Bit of hepatitis" and "Like the flu" to patients, imagine if 90% of cigarette kills vanished, they would still be handing them out with bad tasting prescriptions like the Fifties.

Illnesses Associated with Viral Hepatitis are Booming

Liver Cancer from undiagnosed HBV and HCV

The World Health Organisation estimates that about 40-70% of liver cancers in industralised countries are Hepatitis C or Hepatitis B related. UK figures for liver cancer have trebled since 1975, motored by poor patient hepatitis screening, in 2015 4500 people a year are being diagnosed with this hitherto rare cancer. It is important to remember, first there are 6 stages of fibrosis that lead up to cirrhosis, and then only in most cases does Liver Cancer emerge, rarely with HBV liver cancer can occur without fibrosis.

So from infection until a Cancer outcome takes 20 years or longer, and there are many visible steps that can be noted via scanning the liver and testing the bloods to make certain liver cancer is avoided.

Like most cancer causing virus's early diagnosis is the best chance of survival, but with Hepatitis B & C being carcinogenic viruses, simple monitoring of fibrosis can "see" a liver cancer coming years or even decades ahead, and by diet and treatment can head it off. Especially, if like many you are late diagnosed with advanced liver damage, the HBV and HCV treatments really comes into its own. The line representing Liver Cancer has a 500% growth since 1971, as has liver cirrhosis. The alcohol and obesity lobbies have done an excellent job of claiming all liver problems and funds for themselves. The Chart below was mailed to 300 MP's 10 years ago liver cancer and cirrhosis have sky rocketed while alcohol consumption has fallen 20%, exactly as we predicted.

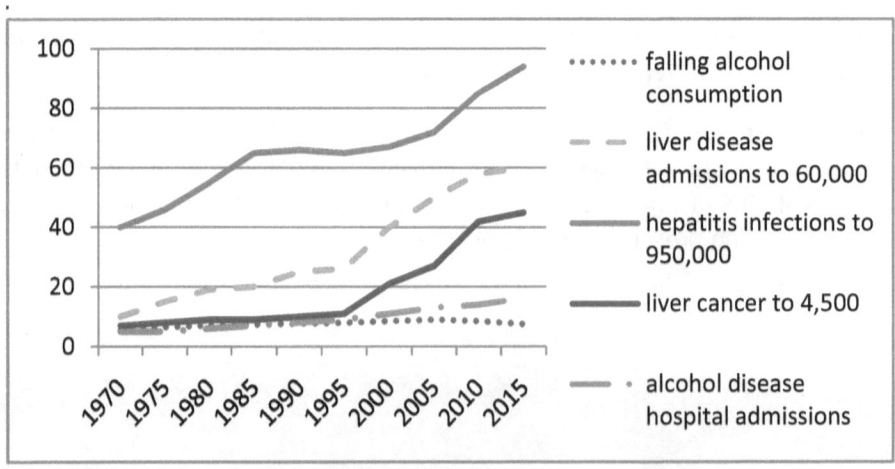

HBV & HCV Liver Failure, Cirrhosis and Rare Cancers are Booming

Bile Duct cancer termed ICC has gone up from 50 a year to 800 a year 1970-2001; again the Hepatitis B and C relationship is high up to 40% in the UK. Globally cancers account for about half of Hepatitis B and C deaths with alcohol/drug reaction liver failure and liver cirrhosis supplying the rest.

Cirrhosis develops in 20-30% of undiagnosed Hepatitis B and C infections. Cirrhosis is a process in which liver cells are damaged or killed and replaced with scar tissue. Extensive scar tissue formation impairs the flow of blood through the liver, causing more liver cell death and a loss of liver function. Cirrhosis affects the liver badly, many of its crucial functions, clotting, maintaining the immune system, digesting, all wane with this condition. Cirrhosis is already present in up to 30% of the newly HBV/HCV diagnosed

Compensated Cirrhosis means that the liver is heavily scarred but can still perform most functions; people with compensated cirrhosis exhibit few or no symptoms. **Decompensated Cirrhosis** is an initial HCV symptom for many infected. It means that the liver is extensively scarred and unable to function. People with decompensated cirrhosis often develop complications such as high blood pressure in the vein that leads to the liver (portal hypertension), varices (stretched blood vessels) in the esophagus and stomach, internal bleeding, ascites (fluid accumulation), and other potentially life-threatening conditions. They may also experience reversible mental confusion.

Alcoholic Liver Failure In the UK we drink 20% less alcohol yet are dying 3 times more from liver failure. Deaths have sky rocketed during the longest drop in alcohol use on record. Our 150,000 undiagnosed for hepatitis drinkers are odds on to experience this. **Drug Reaction Liver Failure** It is estimated 10,000 people a year may be dying as a result of drug reaction liver failure. 6% of UK A&E Admissions are due to drug re action.

To date our GP's may forget to test for Hepatitis, even when diagnoses of cirrhosis, fibrosis, liver failure, liver cancer or persistently high ALTs blood results are indicated. It is also very rare for them to include viral HBV or HCV tests when prescribing liver dangerous medicine or liver function blood tests. So it is important to ask for a test, sometimes repeatedly with the above afflictions. Many callers found GP's had assumed alcoholism rather than HBV or HCV testing, often for decades. One cirrhotic teetotal HCV patient found unkempt smells of alcohol on his notes when changing GP's.

Illnesses related to undiagnosed HBV/HCV are booming

Below the percentages of long term HBV/HCV patients affected by other ailments from published studies

• Gall stones,	17%	Cirrhosis,	25%
• Fibrosis,	35%	Liver failure,	10%
• Liver Cancer,	10%	Poor LFT's,	40%

Overview of Illnesses Linked with Viral Hepatitis

It is important to remember that the vast majority of people with hepatitis may never experience the more severe types of these non liver illnesses above and below. The great shame is so often these conditions are treated without any thought they may be Hepatitis driven by General Practitioners and Hospital Specialists.

Do not let the words scare you, spider nevi are just tiny veins that can discolour the heel! Many of the following are healed by the hepatitis treatment and diet.

The Hepatitis B and C virus mainly affects the liver, but other Illnesses are associated with it. These mainly affect the skin, eyes, joints, immune system, nervous system and kidneys. These conditions seem confined to those having HBV or HCV over two decades to five decades, they also seem far more common among those with high viral loads and high ALT liver function test scores.

I struggled a lot to put this page in as we do not want patients reading this lot and assuming themselves to death, but for many a few of our conditions suddenly make sense.

And ultimately we feel whatever we give the GP's is stuff which patients have a right to. Many callers have kidney and gall stone surgeries to relate at mid life and many experience tiredness and skin problems. The more serious complaints are more among those with fibrosis stage 5 and cirrhosis, we are seriously committed to counting how much Bile Duct, NHL, Kidney, Blood and Skin Cancers are affecting those with HBV and HCV.

Some of these conditions– Cryoglobulinemia, for example – are somewhat more common and well-documented, while others are infrequent or their association with hepatitis has not yet been proven. Several studies have found that between 70-74% of patients experience non liver conditions.

- Common highlights conditions that called twice in one day,
- Speech marks highlight common patient or counselor statements.

Daily "HBV & HCV can affect the skin.""Cause wearying conditions."

Common Peripheral Neuropathy
Common Pruritus 15
Common Arthralgia
Common Fatigue
Common Fibromyalgia
Mooren Corneal Ulceration
Common high ALTs 40%
Cluster Headache
Common Arthritis poly and monooligoarthritis

Increased Sjogren's syndrome
Increased Lichen myxoedematosus
Increased Vitiligo
Porphyria Cutanea Tarda
Thyroid Disease hyperthyroidism
Spider Nevi
Paresthesia
Rare Lichen Planus

Weekly "HBV/HCV affects the veins, kidneys, blood and their functions".

Increased Thrombocytopenia
Increased System Lupus
Increased Insulin Resistance
Neutropenia
Rare Behcet"s Disease
Rare Cerebral Vasculitis

Increased Immune Thrombocytopenic
Increased Vasculitis
Raynaud"s Syndrome
Rare Diabetes
Common Cryoglobulinemia
Hypertrophic Membranous Nephropathy

Monthly "Can affect the lungs." "Can cause non liver cancers."

Increased Waldenstrom Macroglobulinemia
Increased Non-Hodgkin"s Lymphomas
Bile duct and NHL Cancer 1%
Chronic Obstructive Pulmonary Disease

Multiple Myeloma
Kidney Cancer HCVonly0.6%
Asthma
Idiopathic pulmonary fibrosis

Dangerous Cures and Quack Treatments Calls

Into the vacuum of public HBV HCV posters, many fall prey to fringe Christian, African and Muslim healers who often say they have a cure and faith means following Jesus or Mohammed and leaving some or all NHS care. Callers have reported too often communities are turning to their healers first, yellow eyes has created child exorcism frenzy more than once, we had a muslim NHS practice advocate saying Islamic exorcism and bleeding cures HBV once. Islamic, Faith and Witch Doctors practice bleeding hepatitis! Outlawing this madness is much needed, as many see these healers first, many witch doctors are FGM cutters also. Highly priced herbs are also sold as "cures".

Chapter 19 Issues Calls that keep us up at night

Sad. Man and his ventilator
"Liver death is dreadful. We switched off a man on a ventilator today, meaning the doctors, the family, especially the patient had all agreed. Having been on the helpline for 4 months, we knew him well and so we said yes too.
For 20 minutes he suffocated then for 3 he had a heart attack – eternity, all because he missed a HBV vaccination."

Sad. Heamophiliacs are just 2% of those infected by the NHS
"Life is a never ending round of funerals, 2,700 dead, over 4,500 infected," Carol Anne Grayson reporting on NHS HBV/HCV among haemophilia patients

Sad Gran infected in August 2011 by NHS gastroscopy tube contaminated with HBV (previous patient to use it came forward with HBV) went fulminant and died convulsing herself to death in front of grand children in September

Mad. Pakistani Mum Poor messaging and she misunderstood HCV treatment and thought It would make her hair fall out, now terminal liver cancer

Mad. NHS Midwife HBV positive
Admitted having HBV scared as health failing but more scared of losing job by notifying Hospital. There are thousands of views on our HBV positive Nurses come and work for the NHS Web Forum, dozens I have arranged interviews for, where do they all go?

Mad. Lady Told she had HBV in 1998 has avoided marriage and children therefore, just advised by doctor that it was a mistake, a false positive, this is a common confusion.

Mad. School 5 girl's one class with HBV, all girls in class tested. Testing not thought needed across whole school, school nurse not informed!

Mad 12 year old tattooing tiny heart with needle and ink
Said to annoyed mum "It is only tiny, Harry Styles does it, so every 12 year old 1 Directioner does it too!" I mean juvenile scratching is more infectious than heroin addiction and it is on the front of every tweenie magazine everywhere.

Mad Michael Palin having done the street dentistry in Nepal then has a cut throat shave on the street in Pakistan

Meetings that keep us up at night

Sir Partridge CEO Sexual Health Charity asked
"Does anyone know how many people are dying of HBV?" We answered "A 30% confidence interval guess would say from 500,000 with HBV dying at the global .2% annual death rate. We are experiencing entirely preventable deaths every 8 hours or a 1000 a year from HBV and with HCV added at 500,000 and 0.3% as the global death rate we would have 2500 annual deaths from viral hepatitis as opposed to HIV with nearer 250 annual deaths. For a decade all our funding for HBV has gone to Sexual Health and Drug Rehabilitation charities like his. The Terrance Higgins Trust was given more to put up a HBV web page than we have had in a decade"

Minister for Health Ellison
Asked 14 times about our HBV 1.6% infected hospital wards said "We cannot recognize these figures even though we have just printed them." The wards are 8 times worse than the public are being told! Our children tested 35 times more HBV infected than in similar US studies and our entire government is having a whiteout!

Health Secretary 1982-5 Patrick Jenkins
When we presented a one million figure for NHS infections of HBV and HCV post war, he welled up saying the numbers are compelling and I am so very sorry it happened on my watch too.

St John Ambulance HQ
On being advised that first aid without HBV immunity is unsafe with a 1 in 17 career infection rate, St John said it cannot happen and has not happened to their staff. At which point Ian Harmer who is medically documented to be infected as a St John Ambulance man said.   We have not come here to lie. For a man with liver cancer, who has volunteered his life to save others in front of them, who as a undertaker brought troops back from war zones to have to beg he isn't lying! We broke it to St john all 3 of us had first aid hepatitis and truly thousands catch HBV from working with blood unvaccinated. But we still get calls from unwarned unvaccinated St John staff.

NICE For years this unapproachable quango has always refused any member of our strong UK group of patients any voice at all. We still hope one day they can realize the need for representatives of the 150,000 HBV mums, the 50,000 HBV kids, the 2 million in the 14 Industries that work with blood and finally the leaders for ethnic groups with over 3-10% HBV infection levels. Having studiously avoided patients for decades the Institute is still quite unaware 500,000 HBV & HCV innocently infected people exist and are dying for basic very inexpensive healthcare in their thousands.

Maternity unit conference a midwife asked what is the point of core antibody (anti-HBc) testing as they might try it. Later it dawned on me there have been 50,000 mums diagnosed with HBV since 2002, with HBV we would expect 3 times that amount to have signs of a cleared HBV infection or the anti-HBc result asked about. That is 150,000 UK mums who had a cleared HBV result since 2002. Point is all these poor women should have been told "HBV has already infected and tried to kill you" and "The source that infected you is usually just as present for baby, whether family members or an endemic homeland. At 2 babies per mum we worked out 300,000 UK children have a family that catches HBV and are still not told or vaccinated

LBC London Mayors' Questions, announced to the 4,000 Londoners and Boris that their city was going endemic for HBV, 1 in 50 infected with all wards testing at that level already. The shock was palpable, if they could have seen one of the 30 London Assembly members on the stage needing advice for his new HBV infection afterwards. I mean the 30 Assembly members are catching HBV in front of our eyes as I try to warn them.

Emails to sister charity Dr Joan Block, Head of the Charity team that discovered HBV and its vaccine heralded our call to action for HBV vaccinations in the UK. The simple math is with almost identical migrant demographics since 1993 our onward child infections project at 80,000. Medical studies noted that their unvaccinated Chinese children caught HBV at a 1 in 40 annual rate and the US observed the WHO recommendation to protect children. In 2003 a UK medical study noted that our unvaccinated UK Somali children caught HBV at a 1 in 50 rate and no one in the UK knows about the WHO recommendation. I think our children now testing 35 times more infected than US ones, is something everyone has a right to know.

Since 2004 we have met hundreds of liver experts and dozens of professional bodies and all support our call for vaccination of newborns. Yet in 2015 we still as a nation are being told it needs to be cost effective. War torn infrastructure less South Sudan and Somali both managed to work this out in 2013. They were the last on Earth leaving only our PHE punching a calculator for the 22nd year as child infections boom. In 2015 the children in the very hospitals where they work are testing at 0.8% infected and still no reply to our letters and calls.

Chapter 20 Denialism of HBV & HCV as normal and common

As we approach another 28 July, World Hepatitis Day, I am often stunned by how easy and normal understanding HBV and HCV is overseas. This attitude of it is common, easy to innocently catch, crucial to diagnose early and easy to manage is often in general medical circulation, from Africa to Asia, health services and people are relaxed and enthusiastic to promote a liver good life, testing and vaccination in the streets.

Without an "Affects everyone, everywhere" and "Am I the 1 in 4 who catch it" attitude, people are simply not dealing with the reality of HBV & HCV in what is one of the world's most multi racial, multi cultural, globally mobile nations. It is astonishing to think that there are 4 "Infectious Days and Routes" WHO wants every child and human to understand, 3 we know well in the UK

1. **HIV**   **and**   **Sex**
2. **Malaria**   **and**   **Mosquitoes**
3. **TB**   **and**   **Coughing**

Yet the 4th one, the one 10 times the size of HIV and that affects children,

4. **HBV**   **and**   **Blood**

We are in total abject ignorance of. We have failed to teach generation after generation this simple thing, the dangers of wounds and blood, our citizens have no idea of how you get HBV, blood contaminated healthcare and blood and wounds, and they have no idea of the precautions or transmission routes. Of the dozens of media people we have advised of the disaster, Adrian Chiles and Moira Stuart both recognised the scale of the need and both reported our BBC as still unwilling to run a story or warn our citizens. Blood Hygiene, while mandatory on match of the day remains invisible on all child, travel and news programming to date. The BBC is the only national broadcaster to repeatedly cover up viral hepatitis hiding hundreds of thousands of NHS infections, Migration Infections and Child Infections to date. It is incapable of warning our nation that 1 in 3 humans has caught hepatitis, Its politics have gagged it, just when 15 million innocent men women and children need it to broadcast a warning, So we are far more likely to catch and also to die of hepatitis here than any other developed nation. If a national broadcaster cannot say our 10 million children are now testing more infected than our 100,000 heroin addicts, why should it even exist anymore.

The Politics of Denialism

In the late nineties the government of South Africa in the form of Thambo Mbeki and his health minister and their advisors, decided that because the link between Aids and HIV was obscure, that HIV did not necessarily cause AIDS. This decision commentators in Africa have felt was political and motivated in feeling stigma. Whenever a country denies a WHO Epidemic Alert and strap line, it's called denialism. That's because a list of things then happen.

First they deny the disease classification, i.e. HIV causes Aids, then they deny the deaths are related or to count the deaths, then they can forget the strap line safe sex, then people aren't infected and no one's dying and nothing is done - this is denialism in an Aids Context. Historically the apartheid regime also called Aids - American Information Discouraging Sex - some of the Boer's said it was a black disease, then a black and gay disease. Mandela had to say it was a sex disease and found the whites were already 1% HIV positive. A different reason for denialism, but still from 85-92 South Africa had no death certificate or disease classification, and most of all no strap line or condoms.

Now on a global scale, across all sorts of regimes, with 3 new emotive killer viruses, HIV, HBV and HCV, now infecting 1 in 10 of our species, you can imagine there have been many outbreaks of denialism. The UK has had its HCV healthcare impeded by denialism regarding HCV on a unique scale. The strap line Know your risks get tested has been forgotten for 25 years and in 2005 we got street injectors need to learn about HCV instead. WHO classified HBV & HCV carcinogenic in 1994 by 2006 Australia noted 5% of the HCV diagnosed had died of liver cancer (4000+). The UK in 2015 is full of doctors who are told only 300 a year die here. WHO disease classification has also gone from public superbug to a "their" injector problem. Our wholesale prison blood use and 100,000's of infections have vanished. Unfortunately our denialism of HBV & HCV has extended to our borders and world view, over which a denied 150,000 HCV and 300,000 HBV infected people have migrated. Denialism means there is no effective plan for public testing or get tested messages for them or the NHS healthcare infected or our children in need of vaccination.

Or as a globally respected Hepatitis Activist intelligently put it, "Sometimes on the patient's side there's a lot of stigma and shame to admitting to being an injector or a sexually at risk, there again, there's often a lot of reluctance by health services that feel shame and stigma in admitting the Healthcare Nature of the Pandemic." **Chris Kennedy Lawford**

Conclusions

The harder you study the facts, the harder you listen to the evidence for liver cancers and liver cirrhosis' rising to due undiagnosed Hepatitis C and Hepatitis B, the more you feel tens of thousands have died, tens of thousands are dying, and tens of thousands will die unless and here's the rub, we notice.

My point is that most of our liver specialists have been saying since 1989 that unaccountably more people are dying of liver cancers and liver cirrhosis, than is explained by alcohol. If we drink the same amount, something else must be responsible for the 500% extra deaths since 1975. Every Clinician I've come across is dealing with people who they know would have been saved by earlier diagnosis. Hepatitis means guaranteed fibrosis to the 20 year long term undiagnosed that use the wrong household substances. Yet we have practiced twenty years of Wait & See plus a low key Face Addicts Campaign. We are still nowhere near a public test poster or education. 250,000 will die eventually and are visibly dying as predicted, faster and faster.

My point is that when I started this study in London, we had hoped to discover a potential number of HBV & HCV deaths above their admitted underestimate of 100 in 2003. I find that adding the figures up gives nearly 2-4000 deaths per annum, this unfortunately corroborates to the higher estimates of infection levels.

> 2000 annual deaths = 400,000
> 3000 annual deaths = 600,000
> 4000 annual deaths = 800,000

Most of all I've noticed definite efforts and petty arguments to blur the crucial fact; HBV/HCV is causing Liver Cancer, Bile Duct Cancer and HBV and HCV cirrhosis undiagnosed and unchecked in the UK. Having studied the US, French & Canadian look backs at deaths in 99, and their use of the 99 WHO Cause of Death Classification and Look Back to diagnose and protect the bulk of their millions of ex-patients. I ask myself how can our Health Service underestimate a Pandemics fatalities by up to 90%, and this while knowing nearly a 1,000,000 are out there mainly still unwarned and undiagnosed?

I feel like we have found 10,000's of overlooked deaths 100,000's of infections and just complete denial in the air, weirdest of all we are dealing with a globally well documented Pandemic that's infected 70 times more often than HIV! Let us remember Viral Hepatitis kills the undiagnosed far more often. A 100 million of them are dying due to ignorance.

Finally, I hope you have learnt enough from this book to know when to test for viral hepatitis and how to protect yourself and your workmates and families better.

Appendix 1 – The 6 Hepatitis Solutions

The 6 Hepatitis Asks have saved lives for 10-20 years overseas. The 6 Asks are not an expensive healthcare campaign, they are the 1999 WHO Pandemic Fight Back, for the Americas and the EU they are the globally proven 2 decade old best practice. Without them the UK remains the only developed nation with an imbecile debate about the extent of its Hepatitis C or Hepatitis B Epidemics and the amount of growth in their death rate.

WHO Prevalencing for HBV & HCV "Finds" our 500,000 + transfusion infected patients for safety testing.

A HBV Risk Test Poster Gets 50% patient diagnosis levels over 36 months when used nationally and border care safety testing

An HCV Risk Test Poster Gets 50% patient diagnosis levels over 36 months when used nationally and border care safety testing

WHO Death Certificate Usage Counts HBV & HCV Cancers decimating the undiagnosed over 25 years

Blood Hygiene School and Occupational Education
Warns 1 in 12 on Earth and 1 in 65 in the UK bleed Hepatitis B or C

Universal Use of the HBV Vaccine To mirror our mainly undiagnosed 300,000 carriers, with catch up vaccs especially in high prevalence communities.

The Liberal Democrat hosted Party Health Whips Seminar 2009 studied the Asks in detail. As endorsed by Stephen Hughes MEP, EU Committee for Social Crises and by Lord Archer, Chairman of the UK Report into Contaminated Blood. We gratefully accept Former Health Minister Lord Jenkins Apology that infections occurred, and that the numbers we are quoting are "Very Compelling". We request Boris Johnson and David Cameron and all MP's for each Ask. Finally, for 10 years Paul has invested in giving the UK's HBV sufferers a helpline, help groups, research, factsheets, hundreds of pages of updated web advice and a lobby. We have also spent serious time in public lectures and exhibitions and in NHS staff training, yet not £25,000 has been spent by local and central government pharma and lottery etc groups combined to help, this is an awful inequality.

Appendix 2. Prevalencing NHS HCV in Simple WHO Classification Terms

- 10% of transfusions in the US until 1992 were HCV infectious
- Annually infecting 240,000 from 2,400,000 transfusion patients
- 2.5% of transfusions in the UK until 1992 were HCV infectious
- Annually infecting 12,500 from 500,000 transfusion patients

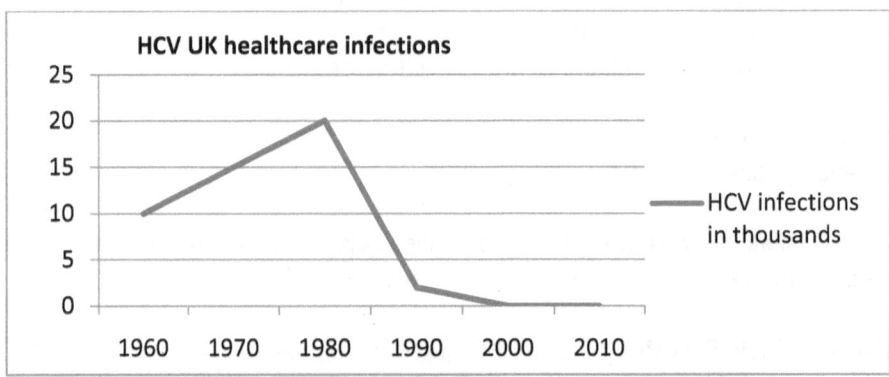

Prevalencing HCV in NHS Surgery Transfusions in Complex Terms

The Public Health Laboratory Service Sera Record below states that Blood samples in 1986 strongly suggested 570,000 UK sero positive infections of hepatitis c [1]. Blood samples also reveal that the bulk of the infections came from pre 1986 NHS healthcare [2] and that Blood samples in 1985 clearly indicate a 1.6% drop in transfusion infections when the National Blood Service stopped harvesting UK prisons [3].

We used about 350-500,000 transfusions annually until 1985, and already have the admission from the NHS that 2.5% [4] or 10-12,000 patients annually up until 1985 received HCV contaminated blood. In 1986 we see the blood supply improve dramatically to a prevalence of 1% HCV infected until 1992. Which is the recorded national prevalence and therefore the expected amount from general public donations 1986-1992. [5]

In the UK between 1986 and 1996 we had some 570-520,000 infections [6]. With an upper total of 200,000 reported for Street Injectors, we posit that the bulk of these infections could only be NHS [7] and overseas healthcare in origin. As posited by our Public Health Service Laboratory Studies below, we are concluding 300,000 healthcare HCV infections, constantly refreshed from overseas reside mainly undiagnosed in the UK.

Appendix 2. Prevalencing NHS HCV in Simple WHO Classification Terms

In 2007 15 years after finally stopping the flow of HCV in our blood supply the UK had the Archer Inquiry into contaminated blood. Sadly Lord Archer had a remit to only study the 4% of infections due to clotting factors and missed reports from the 96% of patients infected via surgery and transfusion. In 2007 to both Lord Archer and the Commons Health Whips, Paul who had quit his Interferon for HCV to be lucid enough, explained total NHS HCV infections.

Using admitted levels of 2.4% HCV infected for surgery and using the Justice Krever model of prevalencing, Paul pointed out UK prison blood had infected 300,000 people with 200,000 survivors in 1996 plus migrant survivors who usually suffered a lot worse from their health services. Where upon the excellent former Secretary for Health Patrick, welled up and truly cared, below in writing I asked him to confirm these infections happened and the numbers are compelling which he did. The key point of the Inquiry is the line where Lord Warner admits we burnt the entire transfusion record to avoid the compensation. Obviously this was done because it was known surgery was at least 1 in 39 HCV infectious post war until effective blood screening in 1992.

Subject: "A Step Change in Hepatitis Awareness"
Date: Sat, 4 Apr 2009 11:48:57 +0100 From: JENKINP@parliament.uk
Attn: Paul Desmond.
Thank you for your letter of the 22nd March, enclosing the papers about the 6 UK Hepatitis Asks. These make very compelling reading, and I am glad to have seen them.
As a former Health Secretary of State, who gave evidence to the Archer Inquiry, I have to be careful about my response to that Report. I regard it as a very thorough piece of work, with some very clear conclusions. It must be for the present Government to reply to the Report and this they have undertaken to do. You will have seen that my evidence to the Inquiry was accepted without question, but that does not leave me free from any responsibility for what happened. Some of it happened on my watch and for that I am extremely sorry.
I will draw your letter and attachment to the attention of Health Ministers and ask for their response, and will be in touch with you when I have this.
Thank you for writing.
Patrick Jenkin
The Rt Hon the Lord Jenkin of Roding

Appendix 3 UK HBV Prevalence 2015 - 502,000

The following figures are easy to reference; HBV prevalences are from published medical studies, populations are from community leaders and ONS sources. The Update includes 5 million newcomers at 3% HBV positive.

Country	Pop	HBV prevalence	HBV Pop	Totals
Zimbabwe	350	9%	31.5	
Nigeria	174	9%	24	
Ghana	96	9%	8.6	
Somalia	108	9%	9.6	
Uganda	60	9%	5.4	
				70,000
China	430	8.6%	40	
Hong Kong	78	8.2%	6.4	
Pilipino	220	10.5%	22	
				68,000
Turkish	500	4.2%	21	
Greek	300	4.5%	13.5	
Romania	68	8%	4	
Poland	750	1.5%	10.6	
				48,000
India	2,000	3.5%	70	
Sri Lanka	200	4.5%	9.1	
Bangladesh	500	4.5%	22.5	
Pakistanis	1,200	3.3%	40	
Afghans	70	6%	4.2	
				145,000
Other countries at 2006 levels			30	

2015 Total for Migrant HBV Infections			**361,000**
UK		0.25%	132	493,000
Mixed Race	2000	.5%	5	498,000
Professions	2000	.5%	5	502,000

2015 Total for all Chronic HBV Infections in the UK

	0.85%	**512,000**

This is not so surprising with the EU average being much the same and our population rapidly becoming the EU's most mixed. However, if we are to import endemic communities we owe it them and their children to provide first world medical care. These nationalities have a human right to public hepatitis information, safety tests, vaccination, treatment and publication of the HBV HCV atlases.

Appendix 4 Status Meditation

One very common problem on the helpline over the last 6 years sexually speaking, is how often people and especially young people have no training in sexual health. Many have never heard of asking a prospective partner their status.

This leads to lots of infections, often people with diseases, HBV included, know they are infected and want an opportunity to say so. Status Meditation is best taught to children during sex education empowering them to know sex without knowing status is dangerous. Because people fail to test their status or lack an education in the value of knowing their status they can infect others.

Across Africa and on the helpline too, we often find once people understand status they can have safe sexual experiences. This is taught globally as ABC

A   **Abstain** until you know their status and know your own, this is love if you think about it.

B   **Be Faithful** when you do, it is worth saying that monogamy increases sexual health,

C   **Use a Condom** when you can't.

All these behaviours increase sexual health and we find empower the sexually active. In Soweto we found this approach, condoms were a day's wages, kept 60% free from HIV and empowered especially the young to value themselves. On the helpline we get numerous calls about when the condoms failed. You can imagine having HBV and the condom failing, before you kill the guy with HBV remember his GP probably told him to do what he has done.

It is crucial to use the excellent tools available; a 100% effective vaccination is always a good status meditation and conversation with any prospective partner. On the helpline we have helped dozens get married and hundreds have children and it always starts with a simple status meditation. It is strange so few have heard such important advice; in Africa mad right wing Christians would ban condoms and here mad leftie politics bans abstinence and fidelity! It is sad so many children catch sexual infections before learning their sexual ABC.

Appendix 5 These two pages are written for Minister Jane Ellison. Opposite are her replies from our Government and Health Service PHE regarding HBV

They comprise the most deadly and ignorant comments in UK medical and parliamentary history.

Firstly and catastrophically the Minister refused any meetings with the infected or ourselves and so was unable to notice the 180,000, 0.3% figure for UK HBV infections is still just a totally outdated guess from 1992. She also failed to recognise our figure for 500,000 HBV infections is based on the 2012 figures for HBV infection revealed by her Department, that we are trying to talk about the 1.6% ward prevalence she has just published. Even more concerning these figures have since been archived rather than discussed.

Although being clearly taught that 81% of patients in our 22 liver units are now migrants she is also unable to recognise they are there at all! Every other Minister on Earth knows 3% of migrants have HBV except ours! Our care for the minority Addict, Gay and Prostitute infections is seen as all that is needed.

Secondly, although globally infecting 30 times more often than TB and killing more people than WW2, HBV is still not understood as a serious infection or transmission risk by our Minister. The pitiful handful of children vaccinated after maternity testing, just 1.6% of migrant children are so lucky, forgets the 98.4% of UK migrant children at high risk unable to access HBV vaccination.

This failed policy is mentioned as if it is useful rather than the reason 0.8% of our children is testing incurably HBV infected on our wards. The Minister is on being alerted to 40,000 child infections and her latest 0.8% HBV child ward prevalence figures clinging to 1992 guesswork data based on extremely flawed blood donation records rather than meeting experts or the children's or charity's representatives.

Terrifyingly, at the same time the Minister is busy archiving without recognising her own reports of sky rocketing HBV & HCV infection levels, our Department of Health has advised her that from 2000 until now there have been only 3 horizontal (child to child or adult to child or object to child) HBV infections recorded in UK children by our entire NHS. Yet in the US just across the water where they have vaccinated all children for 25 years they know they have avoided 500,000 such infections! It is crystal clear HBV is twice as common as chicken pox among migrant children at a glance from the two studies opposite.

Chicken Pox Annual Incidence in England and Wales is 1,290 per 100,000 person years (2005).

HBV Annual Incidence in USA was 2580 per 100 000 in children of Southeast Asian origin (2001)

I mean I often get calls about horizontal child infections, 3 in a day is very common and we have a health service and minister who can say 3 this millennium. Imagine a nation saying 3 for HIV, imagine a nation saying 3 for chicken pox and this idiotic 3 has been said about a deadly very infectious carcinogenic virus on course to kill a 100 million people. We are hearing 3 about a virus that has already infected two thousand million of us, 1 in 4 on Earth, mainly as children!

The last page in this book is still very much to be written by a fresh reply from Jane, hopefully reading this book about herself and knowing hundreds of doctors and employers are using and reading it will help her progress rapidly from the most deadly and ignorant comments in UK medical and parliamentary history, sadly reproduced below, to the 6 Hepatitis Asks and their cost effective roll out as per a developed nation.

Dear David Amess MP Head UK Hepatology Group,
Firstly, the Department of Health does not recognise the figures quoted in the HBV Trust's Report Going Endemic. It estimates that the number of HBV cases in England and Wales is 180,000. The figure you quote of 40,000 HBV infected children in the UK is more than 10 times the Departments estimates. Secondly, the suggestion that the prevalence of hepatitis B has risen substantially as a result of immigration is also not reflected in any Department of Health data. These show that the prevalence of hepatitis B has remained stable following the introduction of clean needles for addicts, blood screening and a selective vaccination campaign for high risk groups.

With regard to safety testing arriving migrants, it is policy to test for TB as it is a serious airborne infection, in contrast, HBV is spread by blood and does not pose the same sort of risk. There are no plans to test for HBV or HCV. Finally, with regard to vaccinating of children born to mothers from high risk communities, all mothers are tested and only the HBV infected will have their children and close families vaccinated. I hope this is helpful. It may be useful for you to meet with the Department of Health at some stage?

Jane Ellison Minister for Public Health 2014.

Appendix 6 GP Hepatitis Empowerment Project - A 6 Asks rollout

In 2013 the Hepatitis B Trust equipped 275 GP practices with the Hepatitis Tools in this book, namely Get Tested Posters for HBV, HCV and Professions, and a Blood Hygiene Poster for Schools. The fact sheets for GP's cover counseling, test results and care pathway advice, we offered helpline, web forum support to the diagnosed. Many of the patient calls that resulted are recorded anonymously within.

Every single Practice reported the Tools were very needed or extremely needed, one managed to test all migrants and another managed to offer all children HBV vaccinations. Proving Practices can offer the correct care for HBV & HCV they simply need training and tools. Too many GP's have forgotten HBV & HCV, or pretend they are a sex/drugs problem still, some are unable to even vaccinate for HBV and have never requested a hepatitis test yet, and these failures are even in city areas. Other Practices opt for a stay stupid until incentivised approach awaiting financial inducements; these always pretend it is just a sex drugs and therefore drug and sex clinic, not family GP problem. We try to get the GP's themselves being from an endemic homeland enthusiastic after saving their families. This worked well.

I remember teaching a hepatitis module and sharing the posters at the Royal College of GP's with Dr Dadabhoy and the point it dawned on one GP he had taken his very young children to two 4% HBV endemic areas, Saudi Arabia and Pakistan for months completely unprotected. They had ritual shaves, tetanus jabs in Sindh and probably lived with other carriers. There are huge numbers of these GP's who are statistically likely to find HBV markers in their greater families and they become champions to test and vaccinate all.

A Practice in Barnes London found offering every newborn combined Hepatitis A and B vaccinations meant it cost next to nothing to offer the service. A Practice in Southall which tested every migrant as per the WHO atlases felt the effort was incredibly cost effective, Dr Ajaib noted it is far better to diagnose people before liver harm happens.

All GP's reported the Posters helped increase Occupational and Migrant HBV & HCV testing and HBV vaccinations. Some were aware leading questions reveal infections also. "Has anyone in the family had a history of liver problems or liver cancer?" and "Does anyone including yourself, remember a period of going yellow skin wise with brown whites to the eyes?" Many GP's quickly noted there are always more infections in the greater family back to uncles and great uncles.

About Paul Desmond

Paul is a recorder who has had time with so many callers, hopefully the book is their best care voice. Paul has run the Hepatitis B Trust National Helpline since 2010, some 10,000 HBV and HCV patients have been advised. The Hepatitis B Trust produces guidance for 14 Industries, GP's and patients. Paul has talked to hundreds of organizations about HBV advising on 300,000 vaccinations; to date his forum has helped over 500,000 viewers. Policy packs for Unions, Schools and Politicians are also produced. Posters and Video's are some 40 more tools.

Paul also has run the Truth About Hepatitis C since 2004 for the 400,000 healthcare infections of HBV and HCV in the UK. Nagging Health Secretaries back to Patrick Jenkins and Lord Owen about the 125,000 plus NHS survivors. From 1985 until 1995 Paul lived and taught Meditation, Human Rights and HIV Awareness in South African Townships. He helped the Charity sector gain 200 million post apartheid for HIV clinics in South Africa.

With 2 nation states Paul has found himself facing a country almost entirely unaware of a blood viral epidemic. In SA Denialism meant the government was lying about the link between HIV and Aids, here the government has not checked for hepatitis in 20 years and still refuses to notice 3% of migrants have always had child acquired HBV. In 2007 Anita Roddick died of a NHS Hepatitis C driven stroke and Paul advised 200 MP's of the 125,000 ignored NHS survivors in her memory, in 2009 Penny Wilson Webb died and handed over the HBV Foundation to Paul to run.

Paul has 3 commitments that guide his work and charities

1. We have to be truthful doctors not spin doctors
2. Best care is based on selfless learning and listening to the infected
3. We treat every patient as we would wish to be treated

Without the above virtues all the medical advances on Earth, HBV vaccinations, HBV tests, anti Virals, liver transplant abilities are quite useless at saving our lives, because we never know we might need them.

Other Books by this author
Going Endemic A HBV Call to Action
Confessions of a Helpline
HBV Accessing Best Care
HBV Vaccination for Staff Manuals
Meditation and Dreams for fairly normal people

Helpline by this author
Paul Desmond is available on **0800 206 1899** at the HBV Trust to help patients manage their infection and also to help Practices and public use the manual to identify risk, to test and to vaccinate workforces, families and educational venues.

Websites by this author
www.hepbpositive.org.uk
www.thetruthabouthepc.co.uk

You Tube Channel
"thetruthabouthepc"

www.ingramcontent.com/pod-product-compliance
Lightning Source LLC
Chambersburg PA
CBHW030745180526
45163CB00003B/921